ECTOGEN

Artificial Womb Technolo
of Human Repro

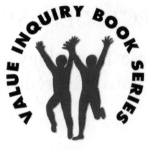

VIBS

Volume 184

Robert Ginsberg
Founding Editor

Peter A. Redpath
Executive Editor

Associate Editors

a volume in
Values in Bioethics
ViB
Matti Häyry, Tuija Takala, Editor

ECTOGENESIS

Artificial Womb Technology and the Future of Human Reproduction

Edited by

Scott Gelfand and John R. Shook

Amsterdam - New York, NY 2006

Cover Design: Studio Pollmann

The paper on which this book is printed meets the requirements of "ISO 9706:1994, Information and documentation - Paper for documents - Requirements for permanence".

ISBN-10: 90-420-2081-4
ISBN-13: 978-90-420-2081-8
©Editions Rodopi B.V., Amsterdam - New York, NY 2006
Printed in the Netherlands

CONTENTS

ACKNOWLEDGEMENTS

The editors are grateful to Charles Scribner's Sons, Indiana University Press, and Blackwell Publishing for permission to reprint these chapters.

"Ectogenesis" by Peter Singer and Deane Wells. Chap. 5 of *Making Babies: The New Science and Ethics of Conception* (New York: Charles Scribner's Sons, 1985), pp. 116–134.

"Is Pregnancy Necessary: Feminist Concerns About Ectogenesis" by Julien S. Murphy. *Hypatia* 4 (1989): 66–84.

"Women, Ectogenesis, and Ethical Theory" by Leslie Cannold. *Journal of Applied Philosophy* 12 (1995): 55–64.

FOREWORD

Human reproduction is undergoing a number of technology-driven expansions, and it is entirely appropriate that we reflect extensively and carefully upon their impact and implications for our ethical values.

As writers for this volume indicate, ectogenesis may prove a boon to women who wish to have children but who have lost their uterus to disease, serving as an alternative to the complex legal and emotional practice of surrogate motherhood in which other women serve as gestators for embryos. Traditional conservative approaches may initially reject ectogenesis, but may find for it a "necessary evil" justification as a compromise between the interests of women who do not want to be pregnant and those who hold that the process of abortion involves unacceptable killing. Beyond that potential compromise, the temptation to use ectogenetic technology may be attractive to women who have no medical condition to address but who wish to avoid the rigors and health threats of pregnancy and its disruption of career and other life activities.

In permitting easy and ready monitoring of and access to the developing fetus, ectogenesis may also evolve as a strong technology in the medical practices of obstetrics and pediatrics. Indeed, ectogenesis, in that it reduces the number of patients involved in pregnancy to just the developing fetus, blurs the distinction between these two medical sub-specialties.

The collision of ectogenetic technology and anti-abortionist movements may have another serious consequence that needs careful contemplation in advance of the clash. Should abortions be restricted to embryo- and fetus-preserving surgeries with the unwanted conceptus transferred to state-supplied artificial wombs, conceivably a million or more wards of the state might be produced annually. The cost of raising those offspring, pegged at a conservative $7,000 per child per year could easily run to several trillion dollars annually for each year's unwanted children. Projected for the 22 years it typically takes for a child to become self-sufficient, and the cost of ectogenic abortions could run in excess of $150 trillion for a single year's worth of "saved" embryos and fetuses. Perhaps in those figures we might find a strong pragmatic argument for a progressive policy toward contraception.

Envisioning these and other practices that may evolve from the maturation of ectogenetic technology along with other reproductive technologies is an appropriate anticipation that will permit careful consideration of arguments aiming at advancing or restricting their use. This book should permit legislators and health regulators to formulate and review policies before the pressure of public demand and the absence of regulation and guidelines result in the kinds of tragedies that arose with surrogacy, in vitro fertilization, cryopreservation of embryos, and other market-driven, inventive appropriations of what were initially only medically-justified technological developments.

Richard T. Hull
Professor Emeritus, University at Buffalo

One

INTRODUCTION

Scott Gelfand

"Ectogenesis" is defined by Webster's as: "Development of a mammalian embryo in an artificial environment."[1] While bioethics textbooks and journals contain numerous essays discussing human cloning, there is little published research addressing the moral permissibility of ectogenesis or the use of artificial womb technology. This is both surprising and troubling given that it is likely that an artificial womb designed for human use will be developed in the near future, and the moral and social implications of ectogenesis are complex and far-reaching. In an essay that appeared on 10 February 2002 in the British newspaper, *The Observer*, Robin McKie states that the most prominent researchers working on ectogenetic technology believe "artificial wombs capable of sustaining a child for nine months will become reality in a few years."[2] Others, like Jeremy Rifkin, are not sure when the artificial womb will be available, but nevertheless believe that the "artificial womb seems the next logical step in a process that has increasingly removed reproduction from traditional maternity and made of it a laboratory process" and it will change "forever our concept of human life."[3]

Prior to the announcement made in 1997 by Scottish scientists who successfully cloned a sheep and produced a lamb most of us now know as Dolly, most researchers and public policy makers believed that human and mammalian cloning were not even close to becoming reality because of technological limitations. Of course, we now know they were wrong. Immediately upon hearing the news that an adult mammal had been cloned, legislators, the scientific community, those who fund scientific research, and the general public reacted with awe, fear, and confusion. Many asked what the implications, ethical or otherwise, were of cloning, especially human cloning. Only ten days after Dolly was born, the United States government issued a regulation temporarily banning the use of federal funds on cloning research.[4] This ban was not passed because cloning was necessarily thought to be morally impermissible. Rather, the alleged justification for the ban was that legislators and the rest of society needed time to consider the moral, legal, and social implications of cloning. Whether this regulation was an appropriate response, I am not sure. But the rapidity of its issuance and the justification provided for its enactment reveals that many were unsure of whether we ought to permit further development of cloning technology and whether cloning technology ought to be legally regulated. Would the response have been different had more study and discussion of cloning taken place prior to the successful birth of Dolly? Again, I am not sure. I do know, however, that prior to the birth of Dolly, philosophers, ethicists, and researchers had devoted considerable time and energy discussing and writing about the moral and legal permissibility of cloning. The response of policy makers suggests that they did not acquaint themselves with the fruits of this research. Given the reaction to cloning, it seems clear that policy makers and the public at large should have been thinking about the implications of cloning before the birth of Dolly so that their reaction to the event would not have been motivated by fear and confusion. I do not claim that we will ever be completely secure in our reactions to developments of biotechnology, but I do believe that legislators and members of society can do a better job of preparing for biotechnological advances than they did with cloning.

Significantly, four months after the birth of Dolly, Dr. Kyoshinori Kuwabara, a researcher at Juntendo University in Tokyo, announced that his research team had successfully utilized an artificial womb to bring to full term a number of goat fetuses that his team had removed from their mother's womb.[5] Kuwabara's artificial womb consisted of a plastic box filled with artificial amniotic fluid into which the goat fetuses were placed. Kuwabara developed machinery, which was connected to the goat fetuses, that performed the functions of the placenta. The development of the goat fetuses at the time they were removed was, according to Kuwabara, equivalent to the development of a human fetus in its 20th to 24th week of gestation. In 1997, Kuwabara believed that it would take about ten years to develop an artificial womb that could be used to bring a sixteen-week human fetus to full term. Others have suggested that such technology might be available even sooner.[6]

Although Kuwabara's intention was not to create an artificial womb that can be used to develop embryos/fetuses from conception until "birth," such technology is not difficult to imagine. At Cornell University, a research team headed by Dr. Hung-Ching Liu is currently developing technology that can be used to keep an embryo alive for longer periods than is now possible before implanting it into a natural uterus. Liu's team constructed a framework of collagen shaped like a uterus, onto which were placed human endometrial cells, which were stimulated to grow. A fertilized ovum was implanted into the cells, and the ovum lived for six days, at which time Liu halted the experiment. Liu states that she hopes to "create complete artificial wombs using these techniques in a few years."[7]

When technology like that being developed by Liu is combined with that being developed by Kuwabara, we may be able to gestate for the full term an embryo conceived through the use of *in vitro* fertilization. In other words, we might soon see the day when a woman's contribution to the birth of a live baby will be similar to that of a man, namely, both will only need to provide or donate gametes. Given that such technology might be only years away and has potentially far reaching moral and social implications, it is surprising that little research has been published on the moral permissibility of the use of ecto-genesis or on how the use of this technology ought to be regulated, if at all. Unless we want to be in the same position that we were in when cloning became a reality (in fact a worse position), we ought to begin examining and discussing the ethical implications of ectogenesis now.

The idea of ectogenesis is hardly novel. In the sixteenth century, Auroleus Phillipus Theophrastus Bombastus von Hohenheim, *aka* Paracelsus, provided the recipe for creating a homunculus, an artificial man with no soul, in an artificial womb. "Let the semen of a man putrefy by itself in a sealed cucurbite with the highest putrefaction of the *venter equines* [the belly or womb of a horse] for forty days, or until it begins at last to live, move, and be agitated, which can easily be seen. After this time it will be in some degree like a human being, but, nevertheless transparent and without body. If now, after this, it be every day nourished and fed cautiously and prudently with the *arcanum* of human blood, and kept for forty weeks in the perpetual and equal heat of *venter equinus*, it becomes thenceforth a true and living infant, having all the members of a child that is born from a woman, but much smaller."[8]

As Rosemarie Tong discusses in Chapter 4 of this volume, ectogenesis has been discussed at various times during the twentieth century, beginning with a discussion by physiologist/geneticist J.B.S. Haldane in *Daedalus* in the early 1900s, where Haldane suggests that the development of ectogenesis would be one of the most important scientific discoveries in the history of man.[9] In the 1970s and 80s, the debate re-emerged, this time between femi-nists arguing about whether ectogenesis would be a liberating or oppressing technology. During this round of discussion, Shulamith Firestone, in *The Dialectic of Sex*, famously argues for ectogenesis, claiming that pregnancy is harmful to women and is the ultimate cause of sexual inequality, leading to an unequal and unfair division of labor that leads to further inequalities.[10] Until an artificial womb is created, Firestone argues, women will not be able to become self-sufficient and compete on equal terms in the marketplace. The recent research of Kuwaba and Liu has reignited the debates surrounding ectogenesis.

As the chapters in the volume reveal, the development of ectogenetic technology raises a host of moral, legal, and social questions. Is ectogenesis ever morally permissible, and if so, under what circumstances? How will ectogenesis affect the abortion debate? How will ectogenesis affect women? Will ectogenesis enhance or diminish women's reproductive rights and/or their economic opportunities? Will ectogenesis enhance or diminish men's rights to have input on abortion decisions? Will ectogenesis allow men to have babies without the help or assistance of women? What laws, if any, ought to be enacted regulating ectogenesis and experimentation on *in vitro* embryos/ fetuses? The essays included in this anthology cover a wide a varied terrain and attempt to address these and other questions. The anthology begins with three previously published essays, which are followed by eight heretofore unpublished essays.

The first essay is a chapter from Peter Singer and Deanne Wells' influential book, *Making Babies*, that was published in 1985. Singer and Wells explore five reasons in support of ectogenesis and five objections to ectogenesis. They conclude that ectogenesis is morally permissible.

The second essay, "Is Pregnancy Necessary: Feminist Concerns About Ectogenesis," was written by Julien S. Murphy and published in *Hypatia* in 1989. Murphy explores the implications of three lines of reproductive rights arguments on ectogenesis. Murphy concludes that these lines of argument do not provide strong grounds for rejecting the use of this technology. Murphy then suggests, however, that ectogenesis may be objectionable in that it might lead to the oppression of women in a number of ways, including, limiting women's reproductive rights and perpetuating the unequal distribution of medical resources. Murphy concludes that a strong challenge to ectogenesis will require a rethinking of women's relationship to pregnancy.

The third and final previously published essay is Leslie Cannold's "Women, Ectogenesis, and Ethical Theory." In this essay, which was published in the *Journal of Applied Philosophy* in 1995, Cannold argues that two lines of argument concerning the morality abortion rights logically imply support for ectogenesis as a means of resolving the abortion debate. Yet, empirical evidence indicates that those in support of abortion rights and those opposed to abortion rights reject ectogenesis. Cannold concludes by arguing that the views of ethicists must reflect more closely the views of women in order to preserve ethical relevance.

The eight previously unpublished essays begin where the three previously published essays left off. Rosemarie Tong's chapter on "Out of Body Gestation: In Whose Best Interests?" begins with a discussion of the recent history of ectogenesis. Tong then examines arguments related to ectogenesis, including a number of those put forth by Singer and Wells. Of significant interest to Tong are the following issues: (1) the possible use of ectogenesis as an alternative to abortion, and (2) the replacement of the woman in the quest for the perfect fetal environment.

Gregory Pence argues for ectogenesis in "What's So Good About Natural Motherhood?" He asserts that until actual trials on animal ectogenesis reveal real dangers, experimentation should proceed. Should primate studies show that artificial wombs are safe, the burden of proof should be on critics to explain why this technology should be unavailable for humans. Clearly compelling is the use of ectogenesis where potentially therapeutic "final-hope" efforts for dying premature babies might succeed. Pence furthermore claims that we do not need a comprehensive theory of rights or distributive social justice to make the decision that the selective use of ectogenesis can be in the best interest of the baby or the mother.

Scott Gelfand's chapter, "Ectogenesis and The Ethics of Care," attempts to address the concerns of Cannold with respect to providing an ethical approach that reflects women's views and experience. Gelfand suggests that the ethics of care is in a better position than many realize to provide guidance to bioethics issues generally, and ectogenesis specifically, in both the public and private realms. After a discussion of Gelfand's ethics of care approach, this chapter examines if and when ectogenesis may be permissible and what sorts of regulations related to ectogenesis are appropriate. Gelfand concludes his chapter with a short discussion of how an ethics of care may alter the abortion debate.

Two alternative approaches to ectogenesis from a feminist perspective are provided by Maureen Sander-Staudt's "Of Machine Born? A Feminist Assessment of Ectogenesis and Artificial Wombs" and Joan Woolfrey's "Ectogenesis: Liberation, Technological Tyranny, or Just More of the Same." Sander-Staudt's chapter evaluates ectogenesis using three distinct frameworks of feminist ethics: liberal, radical, and cultural feminisms. Ectogenesis is a feminist issue, Sander-Staudt claims, because of its variable impact on men and women and the relevance of questions of gender. She furthermore asserts that ectogenesis can potentially benefit and harm the social status of women, so there can be no single feminist position. However, the cultural feminist perspective makes a unique departure from standard ethical evaluations of ectogenesis by emphasizing the moral and political value of mother-fetus intersubjectivity.

Woolfrey asks whether Firestone's quest for women's liberation could be achieved by ectogenesis. Woolfrey reviews some of the current ethical concerns surrounding the artificial womb, questioning whether, in today's social environment, Firestone's vision is feasible. As Woolfrey points out, some believe that ectogenesis would be a catalyst for surrendering the restrictive views of women's place in society. She argues, however, that ectogenesis would perpetuate gender injustice since the basic structures of oppression would subvert this new technology to its unjust ends.

Dien Ho, in "Ectogenesis and the Nature of Childbirth," responds to arguments against ectogenesis put forth by Julien Murphy and Leon Kass. Murphy and Kass independently claim that ectogenesis undermines important social values, including the value of natural childbirth. Ho claims that even if we are unable to justify the moral significance of values (associated with the conflict of values related to the ectogenesis debate), this inability poses no threat to arguments like those of Kass and Murphy, contrary to a claim made by Peter Singer in the essay republished in this volume. Ho argues that the ectogenesis debate can be resolved by relying on some shared fundamental values, that is, values associated with conflict resolution. Specifically, Ho argues that in the face of competing values without a clear winner, our commitment to respecting individual autonomy trumps. This commitment to autonomy, Ho claims, entails that ectogenesis ought not to be prohibited.

The two final chapters in this volume address the social implications of ectogenesis. Jennifer Bard's chapter "Immaculate Gestation? How Will Ectogenesis Change Current Paradigms of Social Relationships and Values?" claims that ectogenesis raises a host of legal, moral, and social problems. No longer will there be a reason to privilege the mother over the father in prenatal decisions; such privileging is a premise for positions on abortion, surrogacy, adoption, genetic testing, and the disposition of frozen embryos. Bard examines two questions in detail: how will such a change of paradigm affect fetal right to life, and how will the parental right to terminate a pregnancy be affected? Bard suggests that given these significant changes, public debate on ectogenesis and the implications of ectogenesis is required.

In "The Artificial Womb and Human Subject Research," the last chapter in this volume, Joyce M. Raskin and Nadav Mazor question whether the field of human subject research is sufficiently equipped for the challenges resulting from research associated with ectogenesis. The authors review the current standards governing human subject research and suggest adaptations of these standards in order to balance valuable scientific research and the meaning they wish to attribute to *in vitro* fetuses.

Six of the chapters in this volume were presented (in whole or part) at an international conference sponsored by The Ethics Center at Oklahoma State University and entitled: "The End of Natural Motherhood? The Artificial Womb and Designer Babies." At this conference, which was the first ever on the topic of ectogenesis, it was clear to all present that scholarship related to the social, moral, and legal implications of ectogenesis is in its infancy, and that further research is necessary. I hope that this volume helps address this need and promotes discussion on how we as a society ought to proceed.

NOTES

1. *Webster's 3rd New International Dictionary*.
2. Robin McKie, *The Observer*, 10 February 2002.
3. Jeremy Rifkin, *The Guardian*, 17 January 2002.
4. *Washington Post* (5 March 1997), p. A10.
5. Reuters News Wire, "Japanese Scientist Develops Artificial Womb," (18 July 1997).
6. Natalie Angier, "Baby in a Box," *New York Times Magazine* (16 May 1999), pp. 86, 88, 90, 154.
7. Sacha Zimmerman, "The Real Threat to *Roe v. Wade*," *Gene Expression*, http://www.gnxp.com/MT2/archives/000867.html.

8. Auroleus Phillipus Theophrastus Bombastus von Hohenheim, *aka* Paracelsus, *Concerning the Nature of Things*, in *The Hermetic and Alchemical Writings of Paracelsus, Vol. 1*, ed. Arthur E. Waite (New Hyde Park, N.Y.: University Books, 1967), p. 124.

9. J. B. S. Haldane, *Daedalus or Science and the Future*, in *Haldane's Daedalus Revisited*, ed. Krishna R. Dronamraju (Oxford: Oxford University Press, 1995), pp. 41–42.

10. Shulamith Firestone, *The Dialectic of Sex* (New York: William Morrow and Company, 1970), p. 232–234.

Two

ECTOGENESIS

Peter Singer and Deane Wells

On 4 January 1981, Faye Bland went into premature labor. Only six and a half months pregnant, she fully expected to lose the baby. She was rushed into the Queen Victoria Medical Centre where doctors attempted to stop the labor. Despite their efforts, some thirty hours later Kim Bland was born. He was alive but tiny, weighing only 470 grams (just over 1 lb.). Nevertheless, the doctors used all the modern technology of neonatal intensive care units. He was fed through a tube and kept warm in a humidicrib. He did not die. At first he lost weight, dropping to a mere 420 grams (0.9 lbs.); but then he started gaining. Kim had his problems. When he weighed 1,130 grams (2.5 lb.), he had a hernia operation. At six weeks of age, he had a leg fracture due to calcium deficiency. But he continued to grow, came out of the humidicrib, and could be fed from a bottle. A year later, Kim came back to the hospital for birthday celebrations. He was the smallest baby to have survived at the Queen Victoria Medical Centre and one of the smallest anywhere in the world. Though extreme prematurity often leads to some form of handicap, Kim was entirely normal.

Ten years ago, a baby like Kim Bland would have had no chance of survival. Doctors' efforts were concentrated on trying to save babies weighing around 1,500 grams (3.3 lbs.): those weighing under 1,000 grams (2.2 lbs.) were allowed to die because nothing much could be done for them. Now it is common for babies born three or even three and a half months premature to be pulled through the difficult early stages. If present trends continue, there seems little doubt that in another ten years' time there will be nothing remarkable about the survival of a baby weighing 470 grams (1 lb.), and even smaller and more premature babies, now regarded as impossible to save, will be surviving.

Whether this investment in highly sophisticated and extremely expensive medical technology is a good thing is not the point at issue here. Some oppose it on the grounds that medical resources could be better invested elsewhere; others say that the number of infants surviving but severely handicapped is too high a price to pay in terms of human suffering. We shall not enter into this difficult discussion now. Our reference to these developments is simply intended to make the point that the human fetus no longer needs to be in a human womb for anything like the normal nine months. Ectogenesis—the growth and development of a being outside its mother's womb during the period when it would normally be inside the womb—is already a partial reality. Will complete ectogenesis also become a reality in the near future? And if it does, what should be done about it?

The period in which it is necessary for the human fetus to be in its mother's womb is shrinking from both sides. Conception can occur in the laboratory, and the newly created embryo can be kept alive for two or three days while the original single cell splits and each cell splits again and again until the embryo consists of sixteen cells. Then, under present procedures, it is essential to place the embryo in the womb if a pregnancy is to be achieved. According to the published literature, there has not been a pregnancy resulting from implantation of an embryo after more than three days in vitro or of more than thirty-two cells. While they have not been successfully implanted, however, embryos have been kept alive for longer periods. In 1975, Robert Edwards kept three surplus embryos alive instead of dissecting them for microscopic examination as he had done with others. One of them continued to grow for nine days before Edwards, fearful that it would die unexamined, prepared it for dissection. Edwards describes it in these terms:

> The embryo was still a speck, only just visible in our culture dish, but for me it represented the crucial stages of human embryology, the actual moments when the foundations are being laid for the formation of the body's organs. Cells and tissues grew and moved, assuming new forms in readiness for the moment when the embryo would begin to take a recognizable shape. Normally, of course, the embryo would be developing in this way inside its mother's womb, but I was privileged to watch it in our culture dish with all its promise of future growth.

That particular embryo might have lived even longer than nine days if Edwards had not decided to dissect it. Yet Edwards himself has not been able to repeat his early success in keeping an embryo alive for so long. Another Cambridge physiologist, however, has had more success with other species. Dennis New has been able to keep mouse and rat embryos alive for about two weeks. When allowance is made for the normal duration of pregnancy, this is roughly equivalent to four weeks of human embryonic life. By this stage the mouse and rat embryos have formed all their organs and the placenta.

Thus the present gap of a little over five months during which the natural womb is absolutely essential will certainly be reduced and may end up being eliminated altogether. This will occur almost by accident because the ability to keep the immature fetus alive outside the womb will not be developed by researchers deliberately seeking to make ectogenesis possible but rather by doctors attempting to save the lives of premature babies. At the other end, it is hard to imagine that researchers investigating early embryo development will not, sooner or later, discover the defect in the laboratory environment that makes embryos cease to grow beyond a certain stage. Why should the replication of the condition of the womb be an insoluble mystery when the problem of replicating the conditions necessary for conception has been solved?

Having stumbled on ectogenesis in this manner, we shall then have to decide whether to make use of the possibility thus created.

1. The Case for Ectogenesis

A. The Medical Grounds

Medically speaking, ectogenesis offers an alternative to surrogate motherhood for women who are incapable of pregnancy or for whom pregnancy is not recommended on medical grounds. As we saw in our discussion of surrogate motherhood, the most likely cases are women who have had a hysterectomy or women with a health problem that could be worsened by pregnancy. Such women would still provide fertile eggs. These could be obtained by laparoscopy, fertilized in vitro with their partner's sperm, and the embryo would then continue to grow "in the test tube" —actually in some much more complicated kind of artificial womb—until it was old enough to be "born," presumably first into a humidicrib and only later into the normal environment.

The medical case for ectogenesis, then, would consist of the medical case for surrogate motherhood coupled with the claim that ectogenesis should be chosen in preference to surrogacy. The reason for this preference might be one of the objections to surrogate motherhood we have already discussed. If, for instance, early experience with surrogacy showed that surrogate mothers could not be relied upon to give up to their genetic parents the children they had carried, ectogenesis might be thought better than a battle over custody. Evidence that surrogate mothers frequently smoked or took alcohol or drugs that caused harm to the baby might be another reason for preferring the strictly controlled artificial environment. It might be that in a voluntary system there would be a shortage of women willing to be surrogates. It might be, in a country that opted for a market system, that the cost of employing a surrogate is too high, and ectogenesis—once it becomes a standard procedure—is a more economical alternative.

B. The End of Abortion?

Odd as it may seem, ectogenesis conceivably could win the support of right-to-life organizations and others opposed to abortion. Those who take this view are opposed, of course, to any experiments on the human embryo that carry a risk of its death; but efforts to save the lives of premature babies are not experiments in this sense. The techniques used may be experimental, but they will be acceptable as long as they give the baby a greater chance of life than it would otherwise have. Thus, those who believe that the embryo is a human being from the moment of conception must support medical developments that are extending the period during which a natural womb is not required. Since for those who take this view there is no point before conception at which the embryo lacks a right to life, there is no point at which this process of extension should stop. They should support its extension to all cases of spontaneous— that is, not deliberately induced—abortion, no matter how soon after conception the spontaneous abortion should occur.

And what of deliberately induced abortions? Ectogenesis could at some future time make right-to-life organizations drop their objections to abortion; for it is only our inability to keep early fetuses alive that makes abortion synonymous with the violation of any right to life that the fetus may have. If we could keep a fetus alive outside the body, abortions could be done using techniques that would not harm the fetuses, and the fetuses, or newborn babies as they would then be, could be adopted—if there were enough willing couples. Abortions would in effect become early births, and the destruction of the unborn would cease.

Would those who now argue for the permissibility of abortion object to this development? If the feminist argument for abortion takes its stand on the right of women to control their own bodies, feminists at least should not object. Freedom to choose what is to happen to one's body is one thing; freedom to insist on the death of a being that is capable of living outside one's body is another. At present these two are inextricably linked, and so the woman's freedom to choose conflicts head-on with the alleged right to life of the fetus. When ectogenesis becomes possible, these two issues will break apart, and women will choose to terminate their pregnancies without thereby choosing the inevitable death of the fetuses they are carrying. Pro-choice feminists and pro-fetus right-to-lifers can then embrace in happy harmony.

Some who now defend abortion might still object that the woman has a right to decide whether her embryo lives or dies. She may not wish to keep it, and yet she may not like the idea of it being handed over to another couple. So should she not have the right to have it aborted in a manner that ensures its death? But this is a very different argument from the usual pro-choice argument for abortion. It could only be accepted if the claim that the fetus has a right to life had been disproved, and even then it is difficult to see why a healthy fetus should die if there is someone who wishes to adopt it and will give it the opportunity of a worthwhile life. We do not now allow a mother to kill her newborn baby because she does not wish either to keep it or to hand it over for adoption. Unless we were to change our mind about this, it is difficult to see why we should give this right to a woman in respect of a fetus she is carrying if her desire to be rid of the fetus can be fully satisfied without threatening the life of the fetus.

Those opposed to abortion thus ought to welcome the development of ectogenesis, at least in so far as it can be developed without deliberately risking the lives of embryos in experimental work. Feminists, too, should welcome it for the simple reason that it promises to defuse the whole abortion issue and thus end the threat that opponents of abortion will one day succeed in their efforts to deny women the freedom to control their own reproductive organs.

C. Reproductive Equality?

In *The Dialectic of Sex*, one of the seminal works of the modern feminist movement, Shulamith Firestone argues that the ultimate cause of inequality between the sexes is simply the natural reproductive difference between males and females. The biological family forms a basic reproductive unit, but within this unit the division of biological labor is fundamentally unequal. Women must go through pregnancy and childbirth, breast-feeding, and caring for the infants. All this restricts their ability to be self-sufficient and makes them dependent on males for physical survival. Venturing further still, Firestone suggests that this initial division of reproductive labor led directly to the general division of labor between males and females and in turn is at the root of further divisions into economic and cultural classes. Thus she claims to have taken Marx's analysis of the economic division of labor back one step further, to its roots in the biological division of the sexes.

Some feminists are understandably reluctant to accept Firestone's view. If the basic cause of women's inequality is the natural method of continuing our species, the prospects of achieving equality look dim. Most feminists are happier attributing female inequality to upbringing and indoctrination, leaving biological explanations to those who say that male supremacy is natural and unchanging. Firestone, however, has the boldness to offer a biological reason for female inequality and then urge us to do something about it. Her solution is ectogenesis:

> I submit, then, that the first demand for any alternative system must be: 1) *The freeing of women from the tyranny of their reproductive biology by every means available, and the diffusion of the childbearing and childrearing role to the society as a whole, men as well as women.*

Firestone makes it clear that she is not talking simply about better day-care centers, not even "twenty-four-hour child-care centers staffed by men as well as women." Such proposals she describes as "timid." Rather she looks to the "potentials of modern embryology, possibilities still so frightening that they are seldom discussed seriously."

Why do we seldom take these possibilities seriously? One response might be that at the time Firestone was writing, several years before the first successful human fertilization outside the body, ectogenesis seemed too remote to be worth discussion. Firestone, however, has a deeper explanation. Science is in male hands. Just as, in the view of many feminists, the development of a male oral contraceptive has been slowed by male reluctance to share the risks and responsibilities of contraception, so in Firestone's view research into developing new methods of reproduction has been impeded by reluctance to accept new possibilities that could upset the traditional male-dominated family structure. In support of this thesis she points to a fact that we have already noted: any progress toward ectogenesis that has already occurred has not been aimed deliberately at that goal as something itself desirable because of the new options it would create for women. It has been justified on the grounds that it may save babies born prematurely. (Firestone might now add that, at the other end of pregnancy, the development of external fertilization had to be justified on the grounds that it will enable infertile women to fulfill the desire to bear children!)

Ectogenesis, then, can be supported on the ground that it would make a fundamental contribution toward sexual equality. Feminists who accept this argument will wish to see research into the development of complete ectogenesis pushed ahead with all due speed.

D. Better Adjusted Children?

For the sake of completeness, we mention another argument advanced, almost incidentally, by Firestone in her defense of ectogenesis. As ectogenesis liberates women from the burden of pregnancy and childbirth, so too, according to Firestone, it would liberate children from the burden of possessive mothering. In discussing the kind of household unit she would like to see in the future when there would be full equality between the sexes, she says:

> we must be aware that as long as we use natural childbirth methods, the "household" could never be a totally liberating social form. A mother who undergoes a nine-month pregnancy is likely to feel that the product of all that pain and discomfort "belongs" to her ("To think of what I went through to have you!"). But we want to destroy this possessiveness along with its cultural reinforcements so that ... children will be loved for their own sake.

Firestone's claim is that children nurtured from conception outside the body will have a healthier relationship with their mother than normal children. This assertion makes, as we shall see, an interesting contrast to one common objection to ectogenesis. It is now time to turn to this and other objections.

E. The Embryo as a Source of Spare Parts

The final argument for ectogenesis will enthuse some and be utterly repugnant to others. It is that embryos could be kept alive as a source of tissues and organs that could be of great benefit to more mature humans.

Modem medicine uses tissue and organ transplants for a wide variety of purposes. Kidney transplants are obviously to be preferred to lifelong dialysis in patients with kidney disease. Bone-marrow grafts can be lifesaving in patients being treated for leukemia. Cornea transplants have restored the sight of many people with clouded vision. More experimentally, the transplantation of cells from the pancreas is being tried as a means of overcoming diabetes, and there is even talk of the transplantation of brain tissue to overcome brain damage and of nerve tissue to repair the nervous systems of those with spinal injuries.

There are at present two major limitations on the use of tissue and organ transplants. The first is the problem of rejection. Unless the donor is a close relative, the probability is great that the body of the recipient will attack the donated tissue as if it were a foreign body. Heavy doses of drugs can some times suppress this reaction, but they have their own side effects. The risk of rejection varies with the particular tissue being used; in some cases the only way to overcome rejection is for the donated tissue to come from an identical twin, but of course identical twins are not often available.

The second problem is that it is difficult to obtain sufficient organs for transplantation. With something like blood or skin, which will regenerate, it is easy enough to find a donor; but to give up a kidney is a serious matter for a living donor, while brain or nerve tissue or a liver or a pancreas could be taken only from a corpse.

The use of embryos could overcome these limitations. If the embryos were specially grown for the purpose, there would be no shortage of tissue. As for rejection, there is some evidence that embryonic tissue is not as likely to be rejected as adult tissue. But there is also a much more dramatic prospect. As Robert Edwards pointed out at a meeting at Bourn Hall, Cambridge, in 1981, the embryos could be genetically "tailor-made" for the individuals who needed them, so that rejection would not occur. One way of doing this would be by cloning, a technique we shall describe in a later chapter. So far as our present topic is concerned, the essential point is that cloning could produce individuals genetically identical to the person whose cells are used to start the clone. For the purposes of transplanting, a clone would be as good as an identical twin.

It might be thought that embryos are too tiny to produce useful amounts of tissue or organs of the size needed by an adult. Provided the embryos can be kept alive until they have started to form the necessary tissue or organs, however, it might be possible to remove the tissue or organs and keep them alive in a culture. Given the right nutrients, the organs would grow very rapidly to normal adult size. This prospect is certainly still some years distant, but it is not impossible that we might one day grow embryos so as to save the lives of those with diseased kidneys, livers, or hearts, to enable diabetics to produce their own insulin, and to provide nerve tissue that could make paraplegics walk again.

This would be partial, not complete ectogenesis, since obviously the embryo is not brought through to a time when it can survive on its own. Its survival is not the aim of the procedure: the survival of others is.

2. Objections to Ectogenesis

A. The Ectogenetic Child

Suppose that we develop the technical ability to keep an embryo alive and growing outside its mother's womb. How could there be any guarantee that the subsequent child would develop normally? Might there not be some thing, whether chemical or emotional, that is transmitted from the mother to her child during pregnancy and that we are unable to detect? Without this element, mightn't the child be permanently disadvantaged, physically or mentally?

Given our lack of complete knowledge of the conditions needed for fully normal, well-adjusted children, any attempt to nurture a child entirely outside the womb would be experimentation with human life. It would be an especially reckless form of experimentation because it would be several years before it could be established if the children of ectogenesis were normal in their emotional and mental development; meanwhile, several thousand ectogenetic children might have been brought into existence, all destined for a deprived human life. Therefore, those who urge this objection will say that ectogenesis should be totally prohibited.

B. The Ectogenetic Mother

Shulamith Firestone saw the special mother–child relationship as an aspect of female inequality and therefore something to be done away with if at all possible. More traditionally minded people might object to ectogenesis on the grounds that mothers are better, more caring parents precisely because they have carried the child in so intimate a manner. The bonding thus begun already in pregnancy continues after birth, these people would say, and is desirable not only from the point of view of the child, but also from the point of view of the woman, for whom the experience is more emotionally fulfilling than any other.

Viewed through traditional eyes, a woman who could become pregnant but chose ectogenesis would be shirking her obligations as a mother and denying her essential identity as a woman. Granted, pregnancy can be uncomfortable and childbirth can be painful, but they are part of the collective experience of womanhood, and no woman can avoid them without feeling a lack of fulfillment, with subsequent damage to her feminine psyche.

It should also be said that not all feminists share Firestone's view that the new reproductive technology would be a means of liberating women. A recent collection of essays by feminists entitled *Test-Tube Women: What Future for Motherhood?* clearly reveals a sharp difference of opinion among feminists on this issue. Some, like Nancy Breeze, still see the new technology as a source of hope:

> Two thousand years of morning sickness and stretch marks have not resulted in liberation for women or children. If you should run into a petri dish, it could turn out to be your best friend. So rock it; don't knock it!

Others, like Robyn Rowland, are quite hostile:

> ... ultimately the new technology will be used for the benefit of men and to the detriment of women. Although technology itself is not always a negative development, the real question has always been— who controls it? Biological technology is in the hands of men.

And Rowland concludes with a warning as dire as any uttered by the most conservative opponents of IVF:

> What may be happening is the last battle in the long war of men against women. Women's position is most precarious ... we may find ourselves without a product of any kind with which to bargain. For the history of "mankind" women have been seen in terms of their value as child-bearers. We have to ask, if that last power is taken and controlled by men, what role is envisaged for women in the new world? Will women become obsolete? Will we be fighting to retain or reclaim the right to bear children—has patriarchy conned us once again? I urge you sisters to be vigilant.

C. Unnaturalness

This objection should by now be familiar. Those who consider in vitro fertilization "unnatural" will certainly consider ectogenesis still more so. Undoubtedly it *is* still more unnatural in the sense in which anything that is the result of the application of human intelligence to the task of altering our basic biological condition is "unnatural." In that sense, even surrogate motherhood is closer to our natural condition than ectogenesis, for surrogate motherhood at least uses all the normal biological resources of the female body.

D. Approaching Brave New World

Here is another familiar objection. If the term "test-tube–babies" was instantly applied to in vitro fertilization, how much more appropriate it is for the embryo developing entirely outside the body. In fact ectogenesis will certainly not take place in anything as simple as a test tube, but the parallel is nevertheless far closer than it was in the simpler case of IVF. Ectogenesis would make it technically possible to mass-produce babies in the manner Aldous Huxley describes in *Brave New World*. For this reason, some will say, we should not move toward ectogenesis. There are some forms of knowledge it would be better not to have.

E. Farming Human Beings

Finally there is the objection to the use of the embryo as a means of growing organs as spare parts. For anyone who holds that from the moment of conception there is a human being with the same right to life as any other human being, the suggestion that we grow embryos for spare parts amounts to a proposal to farm—and subsequently slaughter—human beings. From this perspective it would be the most grotesque violation of human rights imaginable, a form of slavery in which even the life of the slave is not spared. It would be the deliberate and institutionalized violation of the most fundamental of all human rights.

3. Discussion

We listed five reasons for going ahead with ectogenesis: to help couples who cannot otherwise have a child, except by the use of a surrogate, where for some reason ectogenesis is preferred to surrogacy; to create a source of spare parts needed to replace diseased organs; to eliminate the wastage of embryonic life now caused by abortion; to eliminate the present inequality in the division of reproductive labor; and to reduce the possessiveness of natural mothers. In the absence of any decisive objections to ectogenesis, any one of the first four reasons would be sufficient to justify the procedure.

 None of them is altogether negligible. Helping infertile couples is, in itself, a good thing. So is—even more obviously—saving the lives of those who would otherwise die from a deteriorating heart or kidney. Although there is debate over the status of embryonic life, who would deny the value of a procedure that would allow women complete control over their reproduction and at the same time end the present waiting list for adoption?

 Rather more radical is the idea that there is positive value in the elimination of as much as possible of the differences between the reproductive roles of males and females. Not everyone will agree that equality should go this far.

But Firestone's suggestion might receive wider acceptance if the emphasis were placed more on the enhancement of individual freedom that ectogenesis would bring. Women would not, after all, be compelled to use the new method; all it would do is provide them with a new option. If they wished to avoid pregnancy and childbirth while still having a child of their own, they could; if they preferred the traditional experience, they could of course go through with it all in the traditional manner. Since freedom is almost universally recognized as a good, when Firestone's argument is put in this manner, it too must be generally agreed to carry at least some weight.

We shall not offer any opinion on the fifth reason for ectogenesis— Firestone's claim that the children of ectogenesis would be better adjusted. Whether this would be so is, in our view, impossible to decide before such children exist. Nevertheless, the first four reasons are ample to make out a valid case for ectogenesis. The initial task of our discussion will therefore be to consider whether any of the objections offered—or the sum of them all— amounts to a sufficiently serious reason to outweigh the case in favor.

Let us first consider complete ectogenesis and later deal separately with the proposal to use the embryo as a source of spare parts.

In our view, three of the four objections to complete ectogenesis can readily be dismissed. What we have said earlier about the term "unnatural" can be applied here. There is no appropriate sense of "unnatural" in which respirators for premature babies are natural but ectogenesis is unnatural; yet the opponents of ectogenesis do not wish to oppose respirators. In any case, as we have already seen, there is no valid argument from "unnatural" to "wrong." Similarly, while ectogenesis obviously does bring us closer to "Brave New World" in one respect, as we pointed out before, the reasons we object to the society Huxley has described have a lot to do with the political and moral ideals of that society and relatively little to do with its technical capabilities.

For a different reason, we would also dismiss the objection that ecto-genesis is undesirable from the standpoint of the ectogenetic mother. We dismiss this objection not because we deny the value, for many women, of the experience of pregnancy and childbirth "the natural way." Obviously, some radical feminists would deny this value. Firestone, for example, flatly states: "Pregnancy is *barbaric*" and quotes a description of childbirth as "like shitting a pumpkin." It is not necessary for us to take sides on this issue, however, because women are responsible agents capable of choosing for themselves whether to have the experience in question. It would be an act of extraordinary paternalism—never mind about male chauvinism—for a government to tell women that because it knew that pregnancy was good for them, it would not allow the development of alternative means of producing babies.

There may be situations where the case for protecting people against their own folly is so strong that paternalism is justified—compulsory use of helmets by motorcyclists might be an example—but this is surely not one of them. The value that would be enforced—that is, the value of going through the traditional experience of pregnancy and childbirth—is nowhere near as clear-cut as the value of avoiding the head injuries that are more likely to be suffered by motorcyclists without helmets. While no one denies the value of avoiding such injuries, some people do question, and not unreasonably, the value of pregnancy. Paternalism to enforce so contested a value cannot be justified. Women should be allowed to decide what they value and act accordingly. If, as the objection claims, pregnancy and child birth are such rewarding experiences for women, those in favor of the traditional method should have nothing to fear: word will soon spread, and ectogenesis will exist only as the last resort of the otherwise infertile woman. The most likely situation, in fact, is that ectogenesis, like most technologies, will suit some women and not others. The fact that it will not suit everyone is no reason why those who prefer it should not have access to it.

Any state attempt to prevent the development of alternatives to pregnancy would be an instance of predominantly male politicians telling women that they, the men, know better than the women themselves what is best for women. Given this, what are we to make of the objections of those feminists like Robyn Rowland who claim that because the new technology is controlled by men it will work to the disadvantage of women? We can see little basis for such claims. For a start, women have figured quite prominently in the leading IVF teams in Britain, Australia, and the United States: Jean Purdy was an early colleague of Edwards and Steptoe and a co-author of some of the first published papers in this area; Linda Mohr has directed the development of embryo freezing at the Queen Victoria Medical Centre in Melbourne; and in the United States Georgeanna Jones and Joyce Vargyas have played leading roles in the clinics in Norfolk, Virginia and at the University of Southern California, respectively. It seems odd for a feminist to neglect the contributions these women have made. Even if we were to grant, however, that the technology remains predominantly in male hands, it has to be remembered that it was developed in response to the needs of infertile couples—and from the interviews we have conducted and the meetings we have attended, our impression is that while both partners are often very concerned about their childlessness, in those cases in which one partner is more distressed than the other by this situation, that partner is usually the woman. Feminists usually accept that this is so, but attribute it to the power of social conditioning in a patriarchal society. We wonder about this; but in any case, the origin of the strong female desire for children is not really what is in question here. The question is: in what sense is the new technology an instrument of male domination over women? If it is true that the technology was developed at least as much in response to the needs of women as in response to the needs of men, then it is hard to see why a feminist should condemn it.

It might be objected that whatever the origins of IVF and no matter how benign it may be when used to help infertile couples, the further development of techniques such as ectogenesis will reduce the status of women. Again, we are at a loss to see why this should be so. Ectogenesis will, if successful, provide a choice for women, a choice that one can plausibly claim, as Firestone claims, will remove the fundamental biological barrier to complete equality. So where is the danger to women? Does it lie, as Rowland suggests, in the fact that once we have ectogenesis it will be possible for the species to survive without women to bear the children? But women will still have to provide the eggs; they will be no less essential to the survival of the species than males are today. Can it seriously be claimed that in our present society the status of women rests entirely on their role as nurturers of embryos from conception to birth? If we argue that to break the link between women and childbearing would be to undermine the status of women in our society, what are we saying about the ability of women to obtain true equality in other spheres of life? We, at least, are not nearly so pessimistic about the abilities of women to achieve equality with men across the broad range of human endeavor. For that reason, we think women will be helped rather than harmed by the development of a technology that makes it possible for them to have children without being pregnant.

What about the ectogenetic child? This brings us to the most serious difficulty in the way of going ahead with ectogenesis: will the ectogenetic child develop normally?

We saw earlier that the same objection was made to in vitro fertilization when the technique was in its experimental stage. Fears that IVF will lead to a high incidence of abnormal babies have now been set at rest; but this alone does not prove that scientists were justified in taking the risk. Winning a gamble does not always show that taking the gamble was wise in the first place. The only thing that can justify the decision is a careful assessment of the risks as they appeared at the time, leading to the conclusion that the knowledge then available provided a sufficient basis for the belief that the offspring of IVF would not have significantly more defects than children conceived by the usual method.

The same standard should apply to ectogenesis. To meet it may be more difficult than in the case of IVF. In vitro fertilization in humans was based on wide experience of the commercial use of the technique in farm animals, particularly cattle. The resulting offspring had been normal; and while species do vary, there was no reason to think humans and cattle would be different in this respect. Further evidence was provided by laboratory observation of human embryos fertilized outside the body and kept alive in culture for a day or two. Several scientists regarded this as sufficient basis for going ahead with IVF in humans, although they were criticized for so doing by bioethicists like Leon Kass and Paul Ramsey. The problem with ectogenesis is that any work done with nonhuman animals will be less readily applicable to humans than it was in the case of IVF. This is because with ectogenesis the worries would be about whether the baby would turn out normal in a mental and psychological sense—and here the data to be obtained from cattle breeding would not help much. Laboratory studies would also be of little use since it is hard to imagine how anything could be discovered without letting the experiment run its full course, thus producing a child who might very well turn out abnormal. But if it is unethical to attempt ectogenesis in humans until we have a reasonable assurance that it is safe and we can have no reasonable assurance that it is safe until it has been carried out, we seem to be in a classic "catch 22" situation. Work on ectogenesis will remain forever unjustifiable.

Is there any way of breaking through this circle? We can see only one possibility. We mentioned earlier that ectogenesis might arise almost by accident. If we continue to push back the age at which premature babies can be saved, we shall eventually reach the point at which the human embryo produced through IVF can be kept alive without ever putting it inside a human body. We will then have achieved ectogenesis. If this process is a gradual one and we constantly monitor the results of saving these earlier and earlier premature babies, there will not have been any unethical experimentation with human lives. At every stage we will have been doing our best to save the lives of premature babies. The work will have been medical, for the benefit of the patient, rather than scientific, to increase our knowledge—although of course this kind of classification is very rough and the use of new medical techniques often has both a medical and a scientific element.

The essential point is to work up to ectogenesis very gradually. The first step would be for it to become quite routine to save babies born at twenty- four weeks and weighing around 500 grams (1.1 lbs.). We have not quite reached this point, but we are close to it. The next step would be to test these very premature babies at a stage when their mental and psychological development can be measured. This might require waiting as many as six years. Then, if these tests showed that the children had not been harmed by their experience, we could attempt to save even more premature babies. One complicating factor would be that premature babies have a higher rate of handicap than normal children because a defective fetus is more likely to abort spontaneously or be born prematurely than a normal fetus. A higher rate of handicap among premature babies might therefore not indicate that premature birth itself did any harm to a normal baby and would therefore not be a reason against ectogenesis. One would have to try to isolate the effect of prematurity from these other reasons for abnormality.

By this method we might reach ectogenesis in an ethical manner, although it would take many years. Ironically, some of the very people who oppose IVF—and would presumably oppose any direct attempt at ectogenesis—because of the risk involved would think that the method we have just outlined is *too* slow and cautious. This is because they would regard every premature baby as a human being with the same entitlement to have a major effort made to save its life as any other human being would have. Degree of prematurity or risk of major handicap would not be factors they would accept as counting against the obligation to try to save life. Therefore, they would reject our suggestion that before trying to save a 400 gram (slightly under a pound) baby, we should have some evidence that saving 500 gram (slightly over a pound) babies does not lead to a tragically high rate of handicap, with the result that it produces more misery all round than there would have been if these babies had not been saved. They would not regard quality-of-life considerations as a reason for not saving human life if we have the technical means of saving it.

For reasons given in our earlier discussion of the moral status of the embryo, we do not accept this view of the sanctity of every human life, irrespective of its quality. Hence our more cautious approach to saving pre-mature infants and to complete ectogenesis. We have mentioned the alternative view only in order to show that applying a "right-to-life" ethic in this area would, paradoxically, speed up development in the direction of ectogenesis. The overall conclusion is that whatever ethical stance we take eventually there is going to be enough evidence of the safety of the procedures involved to justify the decision to go ahead with ectogenesis. Thus, this final and most serious of the objections to ectogenesis is also not conclusive. It is sufficient to put ectogenesis out of bounds for the immediate future, but in twenty years the situation may be very different.

It remains only for us to consider partial ectogenesis—the proposal to use embryos as a source of organs for transplant surgery. There are internationally accepted guidelines governing the use of human spare parts in transplant surgery. The recognized criterion for the permissibility of transplants of non-regenerative and unpaired body parts is brain death. The total absence of brain function indicates that vital organs may be taken from the body.

In Chapter 3, in discussing the moral status of the embryo, we suggested that if the medical profession and the community as a whole recognize, as they do, a body's lack of a functional brain as a sufficient condition for utilizing transplantable material, then this condition is clearly applicable to, and met by, the early embryo. That is to say, the medical profession's own criterion, logically applied, should legitimate the surgical use of embryonic material for culture and subsequent use as replacement organs or for research up to the point at which the brain begins to function.

Of course, it might be objected than an embryo that has not developed a brain has the potential to do so whereas a brain-dead individual does not have the potential to have a functioning brain. We have already argued against such arguments based on potential in Chapter 3. The potential of the embryo does not distinguish it from the egg and sperm when considered jointly.

We are fortified in our view by the fact that until the brain and nervous system develop, there is no possibility of feeling pain—no more possibility, and indeed less, than in brain-dead individuals who are at present our only source of parts for transplant surgery. Would those who rally to insist upon the inviolability of nonsentient embryos be equally opposed to the use of brain-dead individuals for transplant surgery, thus putting an end to that lifesaving therapy? For that matter, would they be equally opposed to the use of highly sentient animals—like dogs or baboons—that, though they feel pain as acutely as we, are freely used in scientific research or for spare parts? In our view, this is a more serious moral issue, yet many people appear to be more strongly opposed to the use of nonsentient embryos.

We want to be perfectly clear about how far this can be taken. If there is any suspicion that an embryo has developed the rudiments of a brain or that it has become sentient, then it is too late for it to be used for any sort of transplant surgery or research. There must always be a safety margin. No being —of any species—deserves to have gratuitous pain inflicted upon it.

There is one ambiguity about our conclusion that needs to be cleared up. What if an embryo were kept alive beyond the point at which it might normally experience pain; but before this point had been reached, an operation was performed that destroyed the parts of the brain involved in conscious experience? The embryo could then be grown indefinitely without ever being aware of anything. Would this put it in the same ethical category as the early embryo that is incapable of conscious experience?

Here we have a prospect that almost everyone will find repellent: the prospect of growing embryos until they resemble normal babies but with their brains deliberately damaged so that they are in a permanent coma. On the other hand, if it is permissible to grow an embryo for two or three weeks and then terminate its existence, why should it not be permissible to keep it alive while eliminating its capacity for consciousness? To the embryo itself it can make no difference—either way it never will become a being with any feelings. So should we put aside our emotional reaction to the idea and treat the two cases alike?

On this proposal we would emphatically urge caution. If all feelings are put aside, it has to be granted that there is no difference in the moral status of the pre-sentient embryo and the embryo with its capacity for sentience removed. Yet our feelings are not as easy to put aside as such blithe hypothetical statements make it appear. Throughout this book, we have rejected the arguments of those who claim that new developments in reproduction would damage "the moral fabric of our society," where this vague expression stands for some nebulous understanding about marriage or procreation. The proposal we are now considering, however, could do violence to basic attitudes that are more specific and also more fundamental. For reasons that are to be found in our evolution as mammals bearing infants dependent on their parents for a long period, our attitude of care and protection to infants goes very deep. For normal adults, these feelings are an instinctive response to the appearance and behavior of a baby. (They are not evoked by the sight of an embryo—again, for obvious evolutionary reasons.) These feelings are likely to be evoked by the sight of a newborn baby even if we know the baby is incapable of feeling anything. Sometimes, of course, we have to override these feelings and apply our knowledge in the best interests of all concerned. For example, when a baby is born with a grave defect that will mean that its life is going to be miserable and brief, we may decide to allow it to die rather than continue a life that can only bring suffering. To face these situations when they are forced upon us is one thing; to set up such conflicts deliberately is another. For the sake of the welfare of all our children, the basic attitude of care and protection for infants is one we must not imperil. We think this sufficient reason for rejecting, at least for the foreseeable future, the proposal to grow nonsentient embryos beyond the point at which they would normally have become sentient.

Three

IS PREGNANCY NECESSARY? FEMINIST CONCERNS ABOUT ECTOGENESIS

Julien S. Murphy

In the past few decades, great gains have been made in women's reproductive freedoms. Abortion, contraception and sterilization techniques allow women greater control over fertility. Feminists are united in support of these techniques. The feminist issue is not whether there ought to be pregnancy preventatives for women, but that the techniques available ought to be more accessible to women, and researchers ought to develop more effective and safer methods including male contraceptives and an abortifacient.[1] While feminists have been unified in support of methods that enable women to control their own fertility, there is disagreement among feminists about new reproductive techniques designed to treat infertility and induce pregnancy, such as in vitro fertilization, embryo transfer, and research for ectogenesis. If one believes that reproductive freedoms ought to include both fertility and infertility control, it is puzzling that feminists are united in support of the former but divided about the latter.

The feminist debates over the new reproductive technologies which are aimed at treating infertility are very recent. Reproductive rights arguments that feminists have found effective in establishing rights to fertility control seem to have little effect in countering infertility techniques. Yet, given the rapid pace of infertility research and the large number of women involved, feminists need to develop coherent positions that either give valid grounds for making political distinctions between fertility and infertility research, or support both kinds of technology. Central to this task is an evaluation of women's relationship to pregnancy, since the last reproductive technique mentioned, ectogenesis, would replace pregnancy with alternative means of reproduction for some if not all women. Hence, a discussion of ectogenesis is central to the debates about infertility research. Must women be pregnant? Do fetuses belong in women's bodies? Would other alternatives undermine the role of women in society and impede our struggles for liberation?

The topic of ectogenesis is no longer confined to science fiction. Techniques that enable the short-term growth of embryos in vitro suggest the eventual possibility of total growth of embryos outside of women's bodies. Discussions of ectogenesis are commonplace in scientific research and in reports from ethics committees for new reproductive technologies. For instance, ectogenesis is mentioned in *The Warnock Report* (1984). This report claims that it should be a criminal offense to develop a human embryo in vitro beyond fourteen days. This view has been stated even more strongly at a recent bioethics conference where Sir David Napley claimed, "It should be a serious criminal offense to develop a human embryo to full maturity outside the body of a woman."[2] An ectogenetic scenario has been vividly, albeit ironically, described by an editor of a leading journal in reproductive research. Referring to experiments for sustaining human uteri in vitro, he writes

> Transvaginal oocyte recovery, fertilization in vitro, and embryo transfer to an artificially perfused uterus will render motherhood, as we recognize it, obsolete. Women may elect to avoid the disfigurement of pregnancy, pain of childbirth, postpartum blues, and the occasional ineptitudes of obstetricians. It seems like the perfect solution to the diminishing number of practicing obstetricians. Maternal-Fetal medicine specialists would ply their trade on this artificial womb, which would be referred to them by the specialist in techniques of assisted reproduction. The extracorporeal womb could be tossed aside after development was complete. The need for a continuing supply of temporary uteri would keep former obstetricians in work doing the necessary hysterectomies, unless someone should be resourceful enough to develop a method to recycle these used specimens. (McDonough 1988)[3]

Feminists are concerned with how ectogenesis might increase the oppression of women. Clearly, there are other philosophical issues inherent in discussions of ectogenesis. One might question ectogenesis from the point of view of the embryo and ask whether there is any moral violation in sustaining embryos in vitro for either a portion of development (beyond fourteen days) or until full maturity. One might challenge the value scheme in a society that would utilize technological resources for out-of-the-body reproduction. This discussion, while recognizing these issues, takes for its focus the effects of ectogenesis on feminist assumptions about what it means to be a woman.

Would current feminist reproductive rights arguments provide protection from potential abuses of ectogenesis? Some assumptions must be made about the kind of techniques required and the political context in which they would be developed. In order to analyze ectogenesis, let us assume that ectogenetic techniques will not only exist in the future, but will be methodologically similar to and consistent with the current lines of ectogenetic research, and that the socio-political climate of the future society in which ectogenesis might occur will not vary greatly from the present.

Would there be good reasons for feminists to object to ectogenesis? A question central to any ectogenetic research and one that has received very little attention to date: Must women reproduce? While this question is continually raised by individual women about their situations, it is rarely raised of women as a group. Should women, as a group, be liberated from the responsibility of child-bearing? Or, despite our liberation in many areas, does our ability to reproduce dictate a responsibility to ourselves and to future generations to be child-bearers?[4]

Do fetuses "belong" in women's bodies, as *The Warnock Report* and political conservatives claim? Abortion arguments currently do not address this issue. While feminist arguments for freedom to choose abortion affirm women's right to terminate a pregnancy, that affirmation does not imply that women as such ought not be child-bearers, but merely that women should not be pregnant against their will. Hence, the reproductive freedom of women acknowledged by the abortion right claims that pregnancy ought to be a woman choice. But what if very few women chose it? In order to explore the relationship between fetuses and women's bodies, the nature and scope of ectogenetic research must be established.

1. Ectogenetic Research

If ectogenesis is to be accomplished, replacements must be found for the series of biochemical processes performed by women's bodies in pregnancy: egg maturation, fertilization, implantation, and embryo maintenance, temperature control, waste removal and transport of blood, nourishment, oxygen to the embryo. Such a procedure, if successful, would accomplish in vitro gestation (IVG) for human reproduction. I will be using the terms ectogenesis and in vitro gestation as equivalent throughout this discussion. Both refer to the creation of an artificial womb.

The initial steps to develop IVG include the following techniques. Ovulation induction techniques and superovulation techniques enable the control of egg maturation though the actual process remains in vivo. Techniques for in vitro fertilization (IVF) are already in use. IVF and embryo transfer (ET) techniques have resulted in over 2000 live births worldwide, and are a common treatment for some forms of female infertility.[5] Techniques for freezing and thawing eggs, sperm, and embryos have also met with some success. The criterion for success in these procedures is live birth. None of these techniques is completely safe for women and some might be quite dangerous (Laborie 1987, 1988, Rowland 1987a).

Already existing reproductive techniques are pointing the way towards better research strategies for an artificial womb. For instance, it seems clear that a fetus does not need to be implanted in the uterus of its genetic mother in order to thrive, as a recipient uterus has been used in embryo transfer. Also, research techniques for sustaining pregnancies in brain-dead women have resulted in a few live births showing that fetuses can thrive in the bodies of brain-dead pregnant women if there is proper temperature regulation, intubation, and ventilation and all vital organs remain unharmed (Murphy 1989). Neonatal technology has advanced to enable the maintenance of fetuses— some as early as sixteen weeks or as small as two hundred grams—in incubators, though it is quite costly. The longer a fetus can be sustained in utero, the greater its chances of surviving after cesarean section. In one case, a fetus was sustained in a brain-dead pregnant patient for sixty-three days. One researcher, who was prepared to obtain a court order if any relatives of the brain-dead women objected to the procedure, remarked that brain-dead women have no rights because they are considered legally dead, and besides, their bodies are "the cheapest incubators we have."[6]

Other research for artificial wombs uses an artificial medium or even removed human uteri. Gena Corea (1985) notes that techniques for artificial wombs, which have been under investigation since the late nineteen fifties, include several perfusion experiments on aborted fetuses. One experimenter (Goodlin 1963) submerged several fetuses in a high pressure oxygen chamber and used tubes to transport oxygen and nourishment. The fetuses survived this crude form of IVG for less than two days. A research group in Italy has kept human uteri removed from women undergoing hysterectomies alive by per-fusing them in an oxygenated medium. A human blastocyst injected into such a uterus survived for fifty-two hours, and implanted itself (Bulletti 1988). Research to determine the chemical environment necessary for IVG is under way in animal experiments with rat embryos removed from uteri on the tenth day of gestation and cultured with various teratogens.[7]

2. Ectogenesis: Who Wants It?

The research indicates that ectogenesis is of interest to scientists. It is a major component if not the culmination of reproductive technology, for it would provide nearly complete control of the developing embryo throughout gesta-tion. The scientific gains from ectogenesis would be substantial, and it could be used to provide a supply of organs and tissue for transplants. Let us focus on the implications of IVG if it were chosen by women or men as an alternative to pregnancy.

Women might draw upon several medical, social, or professional reasons in their desire for IVG. Whether or not these reasons are sufficient to justify ectogenesis, and what assumptions stand behind these reasons need further discussion. A woman may desire ectogenesis because she is unable to maintain a pregnancy or may have had a hysterectomy. Her medical history might indicate that she would have a high risk pregnancy, or that her health might be impaired because of having endured pregnancy. Other reasons involve the effects that pregnancy can have on women's social and professional lives. A woman may find ectogenesis desirable because she is a smoker, drug user, or casual drinker and does not wish to alter her behavior or place her fetus at risk. Pregnancy might make a woman ineligible for certain career opportunities, (e.g., athletics, dancing, modeling, acting). Her job may be hazardous for pregnant women, yet the temporary transfer to safer working conditions may be impossible or undesirable. A woman may be in good health and fertile but may not want the emotional and physical stress of pregnancy.

Women might desire ectogenesis in order to be freed from the burden of child-bearing within a spousal relationship. Child-bearing has been a blessing and a curse to women. Sometimes, women have revelled in the delights of pregnancy, even finding the female body superior to that of the male for its complicated reproductive possibilities. Other times, child-bearing has fallen to women as a burden. Even in the best of situations, in both heterosexual and lesbian relationships, pregnancy is a woman's job.[8] Finally, some men might find ectogenesis a desirable alternative for it would enable them to have a child on their own, provided there were ova banks.

There are three assumptions that are fundamental to support for ectogenesis: (i) that IVG would not harm fetal development; (ii) IVG privileges a genetically related child over an adopted child, either for ego-centered reasons or because of the shortage of children for adoption; (iii) IVG would not contribute to the further oppression of women. While all supporters of IVG might share the first assumption, along with one of the two positions in the second assumption, it would be feminists who would also be concerned with the third assumption. A discussion of each assumption will follow.

A. IVG and Fetal Harm

The desirability of ectogenesis is predicated on the assumption that IVG would not produce fetal harm. Feminist concern about fetal damage with respect to IVG need not collapse into a fetus-centered perspective on reproductive issues. Usually, in reproductive debates, one must choose one of two perspectives: either a primary focus on respect for women or on the fetus. Janice Raymond (1987) terms the latter perspective a fetalist position and contrasts fetalists with feminists in their reasons for opposition to reproductive technologies. As long as alternative gestation practices require women's bodies, there can be a conflict between women's rights and concern for the fetus. This conflict is illustrated by Annette Burfoot who writes that reproductive medicine "regards women servomechanically as parts of a biological machine whose sole purpose is to nurture embryos" (1988). However, since IVG would not involve women's bodies (assuming egg removal was safe and required consent), concern for fetal harm need not eclipse respect for women's rights. It would seem appropriate to object to a reproductive procedure that might bring harm to a fetus, just as one might object to procedures that harm animals, neonates, or other higher life forms. The goal of IVG must surely be to produce an infant indistinguishable in health and vigor from an infant born of a human pregnancy. Clearly IVG would lose supporters if it harmed fetuses.

It is not known whether techniques for IVG would be safe for the fetus. Even if IVG proved safe in animals, no one would be sure that IVG would be safe in humans until it was actually tried. But who would be the first to risk it? Certainly the fear of irreparable damage to the embryo would be enough to prevent anyone from pursuing the fantasy of ectogenesis. A similar concern marked the precursory stages of IVF. Yet IVF was tried and fortunately does not appear to endanger fetal development severely.[9] One can suspect that IVG, when feasible, will also be tried.

One potential horror would be if IVG damaged the fetus in ways only detectable long after birth. This might give the illusion that techniques were safe and IVG might be used on many embryos before its dangers were discovered. If active euthanasia and infanticide remained prohibited, the infants would be left to a life of suffering. What if severe fetal damage were detected in the later stages of development? Would it be morally permissible to "abort" a third trimester fetus damaged by IVG techniques?

If the fetus were harmed as a result of IVG techniques, one might feel a heavy sense of moral blame. For without IVG techniques, the suffering fetus would not have existed. The use of fetuses in experimental procedures would be questioned. Of course, it would be incumbent on researchers to prove that the fetal damage was caused by IVG techniques and not by defective sperm or eggs. If fetal damage did result from IVG, the ensuing philosophical debate would need to determine the point at which fetal damage was severe enough to make IVG ethically prohibitive.

B. IVG and the Privileging of Genetically Related Children

Does a desire for ectogenesis privilege genetic resemblance? If so, is there anything wrong with preferring to parent a child produced by one's own genetic material rather than a child with a different genetic heritage who might be available for adoption? It could be argued that IVG should not be favored over adoption since adoption provides parents for children who already exist. This assumes that there are children available for adoption, and that the rules and procedures of adoption facilities do not discriminate against competent applicants on grounds of sexual preference, race, class, or marital status.

Even if adoption were possible for most people wanting children, some would still prefer to have a genetic offspring. Is the desire for a genetic offspring merely the result of egocentric prejudice? And if so, is there anything wrong with this? Clearly the desire may be hard to fulfill since human reproduction does not guarantee that one's offspring will share many physical characteristics, or likenesses in character or personality. Even if genetic offspring do not greatly resemble the parent, it is still possible to see resemblances to oneself in the body of one's genetically-related child. This may be enough to satisfy the desire for a genetic offspring. To delight in these resemblances need not be to collapse into narcissism but rather to revel in the mysteries of reproduction.

At what price does IVG offer this? First, this view romanticizes physical resemblances and genetic material. Secondly, there is no valid ground for favoring a child that looks like oneself over another. After all, one's genetic material is so diverse that it does not guarantee a genetically related child will bear any resemblance to oneself. But more importantly, this sort of genetic privileging may lead to discrimination against several groups of people: gay and lesbian couples who are unable to "make" a child "in their own likeness," non-monogamous heterosexual couples whose children will not look like a matched set, and infertile couples, who might expend great economic and personal resources trying to have a "natural child," (rather than all of us spending our efforts on undoing the superiority of the "natural child").

The preference for the natural child reinforces the link between genetic parent and offspring, a link which is often dysfunctional. Such a preference can perpetuate dysfunctional families by social policies that keep the family together because the genetic ties are seen as binding. Also, preference for a genetically similar child reinforces race, class, and cultural prejudices in adoption practices. Families that continue to represent "matched sets" to some extent perpetuate these prejudices in the society at large. In short, the desire for a genetic offspring is loaded with political and social values. Even if our society did not discriminate on any of these grounds, one would need to decide at what point concerns for an over populated world ought to override an individual's right to procreate.

C. IVG and Adoption

If adoption supplied an adequate number of children for people desiring parenthood, and if adoption could be restructured to eliminate long waiting periods, tedious bureaucratic procedures and discrimination, then IVG would seem unnecessary. But what if there were not enough adoptive children available to meet the demand by prospective IVG clients? Should surrogacy arrangements or international adoptions be encouraged? If the latter, it would be important to guarantee that no coercive strategies were used to take children away from their mothers, and that governments were not deliberately negligent about methods of fertility control for women for the sake of profits from their children.

D. Would IVG be a Technique of Liberation?

This question is at the center of the feminist debate over the new reproductive technologies. Much of the discussion has presupposed strong feminist arguments about reproductive rights relevant to fertility control. I believe that an examination of these arguments shows that the oppressive nature of IVG requires challenging the entire context of reproduction. It also raises the question: why are alternatives to pregnancy desirable?

Three lines of argument have been used by feminists to justify reproductive rights for women. The first two are grounded in the notion of individual freedoms implied by having rights over our bodies. They are (1) *Protection of Bodily Violation Argument*, and (2) the *Right to Bodily Control Argument*. I will show that neither can be used to reject appeals for ectogenesis. The Protection from Bodily Violation Argument, while primarily applicable to arguing against assault and rape, has been used extensively in debates about contraceptive methods. The argument states that achieving reproductive ends does not justify subjecting women to unsafe drugs or procedures. Women's health should not be jeopardized just to enable contraception.

Feminists have appealed to the PBVA to protest experimentation with and use of oral contraceptives and unsafe illegal abortions, as well as unnecessary hysterectomies, cesarean sections, and other abuses, (e.g., thalidomide, DES, and the dalkon shield). It has also been used recently by feminists to protest embryo transfer techniques. The claim is that ovulation induction, super ovulation, and embryo transfer techniques are unsafe and medical researchers often fail to inform women about the low probability IVF-ET offers for pregnancy (Soules 1985, Laborie 1987, 1988, Corea and Ince 1987).

The right to Bodily Control is the second line of argument used by feminists to object to reproductive technology. It is commonly used in defense of a woman's right to abortion, but it could be extended to include the freedom to choose or refrain from medical procedures in general, as well as against assault and rape, and in support of safe contraception.

When applied to pregnancy, this argument claims that women have a right to control our bodies in pregnancy, specifically, to choose to not be pregnant. Hence, women ought to have access to safe abortions. Admittedly, for some feminists this right holds only during early stages of fetal development; others extend it throughout pregnancy.

Both lines of argument could be applied to IVG. Feminists could use the Protection from Bodily Violation Argument to object to IVG if the techniques for obtaining eggs for fertilization were unsafe. For even though IVG eliminates the need for women to bear children, it still requires women to supply the eggs.[10] If the methods for egg removal were painful or dangerous, then feminists would object to IVG by appealing to the first argument—bodily violation. Currently laparoscopy is used for egg removal in IVF. Laparoscopy requires local anesthetic, and is inconvenient but not particularly dangerous. Less is known about techniques to control ovulation that often accompany egg removal. If techniques to induce ovulation or super-ovulation are found to endanger women's health, IVG would be a suspect procedure until better techniques were found.

Even if egg removal techniques presented danger to women, some women might still defend IVG as their best option for obtaining a genetic offspring. They might claim that many women in the past chose pregnancy knowing it might very well be life-endangering. Women who survived high risk pregnancies might have found that their choice greatly enhanced their lives. Why then should choosing a high risk egg removal procedure for IVG not be equally justifiable? Of course IVG would not be the only option for these women. One could obtain a genetic offspring by being an egg donor and using a surrogate embryo recipient for IVF-ET. Yet this procedure still involves egg removal and if egg removal techniques are unsafe, women would be enduring health risk in order to pursue this goal. Feminists might argue that reproductive technology should not be used to offer women new ways to risk their lives in reproduction. While each infertile woman would need to weigh her desire for a genetic offspring with risks to her health, feminists might insist that such a wager is not a mark of a liberating technology.

The Right to Bodily Control Argument could also be applied to IVG and egg removal techniques. Both egg removal and egg disposition ought to require informed consent.

An *Expanded Bodily Control Argument* is being used by some feminists who assume that "bodily control" means the right to have full charge of reproduction. IVF-ET and presumably IVG mediate women's access to our reproductive bodies. Several feminists claim that women who choose IVF-ET are reduced to experimental victims of scientific research. Janice Raymond writes that "as women become the penultimate research "subjects" (read objects), the way is paved for women's wider and more drastic use in reproductive research and experimentation. Women become the scheduled raw material in the factory of legalized reproductive experimentation" (1987). IVG might be seen as a case in which women lose all control over reproduction by losing the experience of pregnancy and depending on technicians for the maintenance of their IVG fetuses.

However, IVG might not be a violation of the expanded Right to Bodily Control Argument, if one understood bodily control to include the expansion of options which may or may not be connected to women's direct control. IVG would enable some infertile women to do something they otherwise would not be able to do: reproduce. And IVG could enable fertile women to have genetic offspring without the risk of pregnancy. In short, IVG would expand our reproductive options.

However the creation of additional options need not be a sign of liberation. New options could be exploitive. Imagine a new drug that enabled workers to work for eighteen hour shifts without feeling tired. This discovery, if used to lengthen the work week, would be enslaving not liberating.

Can we envision a scenario where the availability of IVG did not involve exploitation? IVG certainly would not exploit women in a traditional way, by keeping them pregnant. And, as long as women's consent were required for IVG, and pregnancy remained an option for fertile women, IVG would not necessarily be exploitive at all. Whether or not one affirms an expanded sense of bodily control is contingent on how one sees modern medicine, as benefiting or harming health. Women who value the experience of pregnancy and see it as offering a deeply satisfying and unique connection to new life would still choose pregnancy. Women who see pregnancy as either life-threatening or simply undesirable might feel bodily control expanded by the option of IVG. Guidelines for informed consent might ensure that women's eggs would not be used for exploitative ends.

The most extreme objection to IVG might be termed the *Elimination of Women Argument*; it could be derived from the PBVA and RBCA. This argument claims that the aim of certain reproductive techniques is to do away with women altogether. Clearly women researchers are underrepresented in the field of reproductive technology. What is to prevent men from making women extinct once our unique contribution to society—reproduction—can be supplied another way?[11] IVG, accompanied by sex selection techniques and methods for producing synthetic eggs, could guarantee the reproduction of an all male population: the ultimate patriarchal culture.[12] The link between artificial wombs and the possibility of femicide is suggested by Steinbacher and Holmes (1987, p. 57).

> There is no atrocity too terrible for human nature to contemplate and often carry out. This has, in fact, been the case numerous times throughout history, and has been justified as necessary to fulfill the needs and "rights" of "superior" individuals or races.

They suggest that the fate of women might be similar to that of some other oppressed groups (e.g., "witches," American Indians, European Jews). A similarly apocalyptic tone is sounded by Robyn Rowland (1987b, p. 75).

> Much as we turn from consideration of a nuclear aftermath, we turn from seeing a future where children are neither borne or born or where women are forced to bear only sons and to slaughter their foetal daughters.

Chinese and Indian women are already trudging this path. The future of women as a group is at stake and we need to ensure that we have thoroughly considered all possibilities before endorsing technology which could mean the death of the female.

Despite the ever-present threat of violence against the oppressed, the Elimination of Women Argument is implausible. It assumes that women are allowed to exist in patriarchy simply because of their child-bearing function. Despite feminist attacks on female socialization, women's roles in society remain steadfast. Women continue to provide patriarchy with at least four other functions: nurturance, a diligent work force, the maintenance of male egoism, objects of sexual desire. Almost as important as reproduction are the many nurturing roles delegated to women in family life, the community, and the labor force (e.g., nursing, child-care, elementary education, social service, secretarial jobs). It is hard to imagine a sexist government eliminating women only to delegate these undesired nurturing roles to men.

Women also provide patriarchy with cheap labor for tedious jobs (e.g., in electronics, textiles, data processing, and so forth). Women's reputations for small hands and docility make it all the easier to assign such work to them. Men might think it worth while to keep women around to spare themselves these forms of labor.

Further, sexism has been part of society for so long that men have grown accustomed to a position of superiority vis-a-vis women that would be hard to give up. Male egoism is maintained by a sexist culture. Then of course there is a heterosexual structure in patriarchy that is thousands of years old. Male heterosexuality would have to undergo radical transformation. In short, it would be hard to eliminate women if women remained the objects of sexual desire for many men.

In addition to these four functions, women might wage a successful resistance movement All in all, it is hard to see how IVG could lead to such massive social transformations as would be required for a transition to an all male society. The existence of women is built into the sexist socialization patterns of society which requires that women exist.[13]

None of the above three arguments (the PBVA, RBCA, and EWA) defeat ectogenetic research. Furthermore, feminists who see liberating potential in IVG might appeal to Shulamith Firestone, a feminist who has argued that reproduction should not be seen as "women's work" and has advocated ecto-genesis. She claims that "pregnancy is barbaric," "a temporary deformation of the body of the individual for the sake of the species," physically dangerous and painful. Writing in 1970, Firestone envisioned a cultural, economic and sexual revolution which would use technology to expand human freedoms. Ectogenesis would play a key role.

I submit, then, that the first demand for any alternative system must be: *The freeing of women from the tyranny of their reproductive biology by every means available, and the diffusion of the childbearing and childrearing role to the society as a whole, men as well as women* (1970).

Her revolutionary plan requires abolition of capitalism, racism, sexism, the family, marriage, sexual repression (in all of its forms), and all institutions that keep women and children out of the larger society (e.g., female labor and elementary schools). But we should heed her warning: "In the hands of our current society and under the direction of current scientists (few of whom are female) any attempted use of technology to 'free' anybody is suspect" (1970, p. 206).

We are far from achieving the sort of revolution required in order for ectogenesis to be liberating. Capitalism, for instance, continues to be the dominant economic system. Marriages and families although less prevalent than when Firestone wrote, are still the norm; schooling is still compulsory. Yet, advocates of ectogenesis Peter Singer and Deane Wells rely in part on Firestone's writings to claim that ectogenesis ought to be a feminist goal now. They argue that despite widespread sexism, ectogenesis can only enhance the status of women.

Can it seriously be claimed that in our present society the status of women rests entirely on their role as nurturers of embryos from conception to birth? If we argue that to break the link between women and childbearing would be to undermine the status of women in our society what are we saying about the ability of women to obtain true equality in other spheres of life? We, at least, are not nearly so pessimistic about the abilities of women to achieve equality with men across the broad range of human endeavor. For that reason, we think women will be helped rather than harmed by the development of a technology that makes it for them to have children without being pregnant (p. 129, this volume p. 21).

This position ignores the theory of revolution implicit in Firestone's support for ectogenesis. In fact, it would be consistent with Firestone's vision to assume that technology itself would be thoroughly transformed by the transformation of society. Ectogenesis, for instance, could not be advocated as a cure for "infertility," since there would no emphasis on having a biological child. If ectogenesis were to exist at all it would be to create more desired children.

It would be hard to imagine a post-revolutionary society finding a place for IVG. IVG would definitely not replace pregnancy. For if it were to do so, that would suggest that women's bodies had been judged unfit for pregnancy.

Is the best way to abolish sexism a method that downgrades a female capacity—pregnancy? This suggests that the way to deal with difference is to annihilate it.

The sexism of our current society makes evident that we are far from the goals Firestone envisioned. Debates about fertility and infertility as well as research protocols must be seen within this context. As long as egg removal does not produce severe and immediate harm to women, no doubt many will pursue ectogenesis as an alternative to pregnancy. However, while there may be valid reasons for women to seek alternatives to pregnancy, we need to consider possible detrimental effects of the availability of ectogenesis on abortion and pregnancy rights.

IVG endangers abortion rights because the fetus is not inside a woman; hence it would most likely be seen as a patient. (One benefit of IVG is that any treatment for the fetus would not require surgery on its mother.) The IVG-fetus would be a patient that was not (yet) a human being. The IVG fetus, though a patient, and even viable, would not be a person.

If IVG fetuses are not dependent on women's bodies, they may seem to differ only slightly from neonates. Hence, if neonates are persons, why not IVG fetuses too? And what is the moral difference between an IVG fetus and an in utero one?

IVG could thus make it more difficult to justify elective abortions for pregnant women. With IVG, the thorny problem of fetal viability appears. If the definition from *Roe v Wade* remains unchanged, then every IVG-fetus is a viable fetus for viability means the ability to survive outside the mother's womb possibly aided by life-support technology. An IVG-fetus would be viable in all stages of gestation provided it were able to thrive. Hence viability would no longer be a useful indicator of fetal development. Some other criterion would be needed if the fetus were to increase in status as birth approached. The tendency might be to discredit the notion of viability altogether, and prohibit abortion. For if IVG parents went to great expense to reproduce in this manner, they might be less sensitive to pregnant women who wanted to abort healthy fetuses. Should prospective parents of an IVG fetus have the right to terminate the fetus if they wish? This act, similar to an abortion, might be difficult to justify since IVG procedures do not conflict with a woman's right to control her body. The right over genetic material might be included in the overriding right to control one's body. It would be a right for both women and men and so a way of resolving conflicting desires between the two gamete donors would be needed. While this right might justify termination of IVG fetuses, it could also be used by men to demand abortion on the part of their female partners.

IVG could also be implicated in efforts to place greater controls on pregnant women. First, pregnancy might come to be viewed as an inferior act. Women choosing pregnancy over IVG, especially if the latter promised ideal conditions for fetal development, might be seen as taking unnecessary risks with fetal life in order to have an experience of childbirth. Or pregnant women might feel the need to monitor their pregnancies and limit their lives in an attempt to duplicate as much as possible IVG conditions. We might come to see pregnancy as a mere biological function, repeatable in IVG, and not also as a human bond in formation of new life that can be had in no other way. We would need to decide, as a society, whether pregnancy per se, had any intrinsic value. If not, we might judge the ideal conditions for fetal development and freedom from risk for women to outweigh *any* value for pregnancy. Hence, IVG could lead to the creation of a class system in reproduction with the rich reproducing in ectogenic labs while the poor continue to rely on women's bodies for pregnancy.

IVG might also contribute to excessive concern for "quality control" in fetal development. Sex-identification techniques are already in use on some embryos prior to implantation. Genetic research is under way for screening techniques to identify gene-linked traits. If IVG were advocated because it offered ideal conditions for fetal development, it would be hard to imagine researchers resisting the opportunity to ensure ideal fetal quality, despite the fact that such product-control endeavors might undermine respect for life's diversity. In fact, it is the opportunity for genetic engineering that has been seen as one of the greatest dangers of this research (Bradish 1987, Minden 1987, Bullard 1987). Linda Bullard claims that genetic engineering is "inherently Eugenic in that it always requires someone to decide what is a good and a bad gene" (1987, p. 117). We might be able to develop a feminist criterion for genetic engineering, however, such as restricting choices to the prevention of genetic disease (e.g., Down's syndrome, muscular dystrophy, spina bifida, thalassaemia).

E. Is Infertility a Feminist Issue?

Any feminist protest of IVG is likely to be seen as undermining the rights of infertile women to have appropriate medical treatment. What is not obvious is the sexist paradigm assumed by IVG.

This is the most important criticism of IVG for feminists. While those who desire IVG might attempt to justify the procedure on an individual basis, one must also examine the male paradigm of reproduction that any IVG research must assume. The feminist movement ought not to choose sides over which women's rights to support: those of fertile or infertile women. Nor is it appropriate to denigrate those women who choose IVG by assuming they desperately seek motherhood because they are "unenlightened" about their socialization to be mothers. This approach might be plausible if feminists, in large numbers, refuse pregnancy and motherhood as a mark of enlightenment.

However, this is not the case. Given this context, it is unfair for a feminist who has chosen pregnancy or who merely admits to valuing pregnancy, to find an infertile woman's desire to reproduce indicative of patriarchal socialization. This does not mean that other reasons do not exist for condemning IVG. Before going any further, we must consider whether infertility is a disability at all.

Some advocates of reproductive technology argue that infertility is a disability and ought to be treated. Deanne Wells claims, "Prima facie the inability to bring into the world one's own genetic children is a disability in the same way as is short sightedness" (1987). Wells argues that the same objections to the cost and research for infertility treatments could have been made about treatment for shortsightedness in times before the manufacturing of spectacles was discovered. Just as it would seem to object to treating short sightedness, it would similarly be foolish to object to treating infertility. Yet, one should not lose sight of an obvious difference between a reproductive impairment and a visual impairment. The major difference is that while everyone surely desires to have greater visual abilities, not everyone desires to reproduce. Hence, a reproductive impairment need not require treatment. Reproductive abilities, unlike visual abilities, are used seldom in our lives, particularly in the U.S. where the birth rate continues to decrease.

There is another difficulty feminists might have in casting infertility as a "disability." Infertility is a social and political phenomenon. Pregnancy is linked to the essence of being female. Infertility ought not to mark women for the whole of our lives in any primary way.

Nonetheless, women who are unable to reproduce have the right to pursue medical options. Feminist concerns about infertility options ought to center on whether or not infertility treatments restore or replace women's reproductive capacities.

It is imperative to consider the broader implications for women's status of any medical treatment for infertility beyond the actual restoration of women's reproductive functions. IVF-ET for example, could be seen as a new way of legitimating pregnancy as women's social "duty."[14] IVG breaks the necessary connection between women and reproduction, but could imply that pregnancy is merely a collection of bodily processes undermining the reproductive work women do in society. This is not to say that infertility should not be treated. It is merely to say that one should not be short-sighted about the broader social effects of new reproductive methods.

It is not that feminists should not support infertility research. Rather, we should demand a share in controlling its direction. If feminists are going to protest IVG and its precursory techniques (IVF-ET), then we ought also to support research into the causes of infertility. After all, approximately ten per cent of heterosexual couples in the United States are infertile, and most likely that number will increase with the growing number of environmental and reproductive hazards we are exposed to.

The issue then for society and for feminists ought not to be replacing the functions of women's bodies by technological alternatives, but rather developing non-exploitative ways to treat infertility that enable women to experience pregnancy and childbirth. Technology that is restorative, that enables women to experience our reproductive bodies without endangering our health is the sort of technology that feminists can support in a unified way.

Of all the reproductive techniques, ectogenesis, because it could eliminate pregnancy, poses the greatest challenge to women's reproductive rights. There appears to be nothing a priori that requires human gestation to occur in vivo anymore than there is an unwritten law requiring sex be the only means for egg fertilization. But in a patriarchal society we can expect the methods of infertility treatment to reflect sexist biases. IVG does this by suggesting that the way to treat infertility is to remove reproduction from women's bodies completely. Not only does IVG displace our bodily abilities, but it also suggests that gestation in a laboratory is equivalent to human pregnancy. Hence, what women contribute to their pregnancies is not essential to reproduction. Sexism proclaims pregnancy to be "inferior" and men recoil in fear of women's reproductive potential; such are the consequences when those in power do not themselves have such powers.

Clearly, many feminists would favor pregnancy over IVG in most cases, not because women are the most cost-effective uteri (what sort of artificial uterus could also hold down a job and run a family while maintaining a fetus?) but because IVG represents a misguided approach to infertility. That some women might prefer gestation of their fertilized eggs in a laboratory rather than in their own bodies is more of a mark of the oppressive ways in which women's bodies and pregnancy are seen in this culture rather than a sign of progressive social attitudes.

The oppression that leads to such negative attitudes can only be changed by redirecting our priorities. We must ensure that everyone be provided with appropriate health care, as well as other prerequisites for health such as education and decent housing. The effects of poverty on women (not to mention children) are far more devastating than the effects of either infertility or reproductive technology.

We need a woman-centered reproductive agenda that makes visible the needs of all women, particularly poor women and women of color. We are only beginning to realize what this might mean. Without such an agenda, women will continue to be exploited by the sexist research system that is a product of our sexist society. More and more resources, including women's bodies, eggs, and uteri, will be wasted on experiments that undermine women, while social programs that would provide a better life will continue to be neglected. These considerations suggest that feminists must protest sexist research methods such as IVG and politicize not only those most likely to use IVG, but also those most likely not to need it.

NOTES

1. RU486 is the abortifacient currently used in France and is at the center of controversy in the U.S. See Mary Suh (1989) and Victor Navasky (1988).

2. Sir David Napley, past president of the English Law Society, suggested at the 1983 Mogul International Management Consultants Ltd Conference on Bioethics and Law of Human Conception in Vitro. See M. D. Kirby (1984).

3. My thanks to Becky Holmes for bringing this finding to my attention.

4. See Allen (1984).

5. Cf. Patricia Spallone and Deborah Lynn Steinberg (1987) for a survey of IVF research in sixteen countries.

6. Conversations with medical researchers engaged in sustaining pregnancies in brain-dead pregnant women. See Murphy (1989).

7. Cf. Daston (1987).

8. Of course, in lesbian relationships both women can decide together which would "prefer" to have a child, provided both are fertile. While a lesbian relationship model removes some of the automatic "burden," (it is not assumed that one person instead of the other must be the one to be pregnant), still lesbians along with heterosexual women may wish that women could be spared pregnancy.

9. In one 1985 study by the National Perinatal Institute cited in Spallone and Steinberg (1987). IVF infants had a higher incidence of premature births, were four times more likely to die at birth due to prematurity, and the rate of deformed IVF babies was 2.6 percent.

10. See my article (1984) for a discussion of the sexist language of egg removal in medial research.

11. IVG would be the second to the last technique in the series. The final technique might be the manufacture of synthetic eggs, which would enable a perpetual supply of eggs.

12. Cf. Holmes and Hoskins (1987) for feminist critique of sex selection techniques.

13. It might be possible to have an "all male" society while still allowing those of us with female bodies to exist. This would be possible if the category "woman" could be destroyed without requiring the destruction of the category "man." This would assume that masculinity could survive without femininity. The society would be thoroughly masculine in its values. Everyone would be regarded as "men," though some would donate to IVG procedures while others provided sperm. For this to come about women would have to be coerced to take on all the traits of masculinity and would come to be regarded not as a different gender, but rather as inferior men (undesirable mutations of men). This strategy finds limited expression in the world of business and other male-dominated professions.

14. See Crowe (1987) and Solomon (1988).

WORKS CITED

Allen, Jeffner. (1984) "Motherhood: The Annihilation of Women." In *Mothering: Essays in Feminist Theory*, ed. Joyce Trebilcot (New Jersey: Rowman & Allenheld), pp. 315–330.

Arditti, Rita, Renate Duelli Klein, and Shelley Minden, eds. (1984) *Test-tube Women*. London: Pandora Press.

Bulletti, C., V. M. Jasonni, S. Tabanelli, et al. (1988) "Early Human Pregnancy in vitro Utilizing an Artificially Perfused Uterus." *Fertility and Sterility* 49:6 (June), pp. 991–996.

Bradish, Paula. (1987) "From Genetic Counseling and Genetic Analysis, to Genetic Ideal and Genetic Fate." In *Made to Order*. See Spallone (1987).

Bullard, Linda. (1987) "Killing Us Softly: Toward a Feminist Analysis of Genetic Engineering." In *Made to Order*. See Spallone (1987).

Burfoot, Annette. (1988) "A Review of the Third Annual Meeting of the European Society of Human Reproduction and Embryology." *Reproductive and Genetic Engineering* 1:1, pp. 107–111.

Corea, Gena. (1985) *The Mother Machine: Reproductive Technologies from Artificial Insemination to Artificial Wombs*. New York: Harper and Row.

Corea, Gena, J. Hammer, B. Hoskins, J. Raymond, et al. (1987) *Man-made Women: How New Reproductive Technologies Affect Women*. Bloomington: Indiana University Press.

Corea, Gena, and Susan Ince. (1987) "Report of a Survey of IVF Clinics in the U.S." In *Made to Order*. See Spallone (1987).

Crowe, Christine. (1987) "Women Want It: In Vitro Fertilization and Women's Motivations for Participation." In *Made to Order*. See Spallone (1987).

Daston, O. P., M. T. Ebron, B. Carver, et al. (1987) "In vitro Teratogenicity of Ethylenethiourea in the Rat." *Teratology* 35:2, pp. 239–245.

Firestone, Shulamith. (1970) *The Dialectic of Sex*. New York: Bantam.

Goodlin, Robert C. (1963) "An Improved Fetal Incubator." *Transactions of the American Society for Artificial Internal Organs* 9, pp. 348–350.

Holmes, Helen B., and Betty B. Hoskins. (1987) "Prenatal and Preconception Sex Choice Technologies: A Path to Femicide." In *Man-made Women*. See Corea (1987).

Kirby, M. D. (1984) "Bioethics of IVF—The State of the Debate." *Journal of Medical Ethics* 10 (March), pp. 45–48.

Laborie, Françoise. (1987) "Looking for Mothers You Only Find Fetuses." In *Made to Order*. See Spallone (1987).

———. (1988) "New Reproductive Technologies: News from France and Elsewhere." *Reproductive and Genetic Engineering* 1:1, pp. 77–85.

McDonough, Paul G. (1988) "Comment." *Fertility and Sterility* 50:6 (June) 1001–1002.

Minden, Shelley. "Patriarchical Designs: The Genetic Engineering of Human Embryos." In *Made to Order*. See Spallone (1987).

Murphy, Julien S. (1984) "Egg Farming and Women's Future." In *Test-tube Women*, eds. Rita Arditti, Renate Duelli Klein, and Shelley Minden (London: Pandora Press), pp. 65–75.

Murphy, Julien S. (1986) "Abortion Rights and Fetal Termination." *Journal of Social Philosophy* 17 (Winter), pp. 11–15.

Murphy, Julien S. (1989) "Should Pregnancy be Sustained in Brain-dead Women: A Philosophical Discussion of Postmortem Pregnancy." In *Healing Technology: Feminist Perspectives*, ed. Kathryn Strother Ratcliffe (Ann Arbor: University of Michigan Press), pp. 135–159.

Navasky, Victor. (1988) "Bitter Pill." *The Nation* 247:15 (21 November), pp. 515–516.

Raymond, Janice. (1987a) "Fetalists and Feminists: They Are Not the Same." In *Made to Order*. See Spallone (1987).

Rowland, Robyn. (1987a) "Of Women Born, But For How Long? The Relationship of Women to the New Reproductive Technologies and the Issue of Choice. In *Made to Order*. See Spallone (1987).

———. (1987b) "Motherhood, Patriarchal Power, Alienation and the Issue of 'Choice' in Sex Preselection." In *Man-made Women*. See Corea (1987).

Singer, Peter, and Deane Wells. (1985) *Making Babies: The New Science and Ethics of Reproduction*. New York: Charles Scribner's Sons.

Solomon, Alison. (1988) "Integrating Infertility Crisis Counseling into Feminist Practice." *Reproductive and Genetic Engineering* 1:1, pp. 41–49.

Soules, Michael. (1985) "The In Vitro Fertilization Pregnancy Rate—Let's Be Honest with One Another." *Fertility and Sterility* 43:4 (April), pp. 511–513.

Spallone, Patricia and Deborah Lynn Steinberg. (1987) *Made to Order: The Myth of Reproductive and Genetic Progress.* Oxford: Oxford University Press.

Steinbacher, Roberta, and Helen B Holmes. (1987) "Sex Choice Survival and Sisterhood." In *Man-made Women.* See Corea et al. (1987).

Suh, Mary. (1989) "RU Detour." *Ms* (January/February), pp. 135–136.

Warnock, Mary. (1984) *A Question of Life: The Warnock Report on Human Fertilization and Embryology.* Oxford: Basil Blackwell.

Wells, Deane. (1987) "Ectogenesis, Justice and Utility: A Reply to James." *Bioethics* 1:4 (October), pp. 372–379.

Four

WOMEN, ECTOGENESIS, AND ETHICAL THEORY

Leslie Cannold

Current medical advances in the area of infertility medicine and neonatology have made total ectogenesis (the gestation of a human being entirely outside the body of a human female) less a figment of the imagination of science fiction fantasy writers and more a realistic possibility for those living in the not so distant future. Partial ectogenesis is already a reality, as demonstrated by the creation and short-term gestation of embryos in vitro, and the gestation of premature babies in incubators. These developments pose a challenge to several influential philosophical theories on abortion which have presumed that abortion is synonymous with fetal death; a presumption which has and will continue to be challenged by the fast pace of medical development in the areas of infertility medicine and neonatology.

A logical reading of two influential abortion theories, which I shall call "Severance" and "Right to Life," leads to the conclusion that adherents of each would favor the introduction of ectogenetic technology as providing remedies for the aspects of abortion they deem problematic. In fact, a number of Severance ethicists who have anticipated the advent of ectogenesis have overtly stated their commitment to the technology.

Despite the positive attitude of ethicists towards ectogenesis, the results of qualitative research suggest that women's response to the technology would be overwhelmingly negative. This negative response was found in women who described themselves as favoring abortion rights, as well as women who said they opposed abortion rights.[1] The bulk of this paper seeks to describe the moral framework within which the women interviewed considered the morality of abortion; a framework that makes coherent the nearly unanimous rejection of women in the study of ectogenesis as a moral solution to abortion. The lack of "fit" between women's abortion framework and the framework of Severance and Right to Life theorists suggests the need for a reconceptualization of the latter, if ethical theory is to become relevant to women's moral needs.

Firstly, however, a brief look will be taken at the current state of ectogenetic technology, and the evidence available regarding possible advances in the area in the near future. Secondly, the precise nature of Severance and Right to Life abortion theory, and the logically necessary commitment of these theories to ectogenesis as a solution to the abortion conflict, will be explicated. Thirdly, the methodology used in the study will be described.

1. The Reality of Ectogenesis

Infertility technology like IVF and the lowering age of viability[2] have already
made ectogenesis a limited reality. The knowledge necessary for very early ex
utero human development has been and will continue to be acquired by
scientists working towards increasing the success rates of IVF and related
infertility technologies. Current efforts in this area are directed towards improving the culture fluids in which embryos are created and gestated, in order
to increase the number of viable embryos suitable for use in infertility
treatment. While the intent of this experimentation is directed towards higher
IVF success rates, it is clear that the knowledge gained could also be applied to
sustaining very early human development in vitro with the goal of partial or
total ectogenesis.

On the other end of the gestational continuum are the neonatal intensive
care units across the developed world that bring premature babies to term
inside high tech incubators (or ectogenetic wombs); babies whose prospects of
life were minimal only a few decades ago. Whereas twenty years ago little
could be done for babies born under 1000g, today doctors are able to ensure
the survival[3] of many infants born weighing only 500 grams, or just 23 weeks
old.[4] Some neonatologists have suggested that over the next decade, it will
become possible to ensure the survival of babies born after only 16 to 18
weeks in the maternal womb.[5]

Moreover, while funding is not made available in many countries to
scientists working directly on the development of ectogenetic technology, there
are some exceptions to this trend. In 1988, for example, a group of Italian
scientists reported their successful incubation of an embryo for 52 hours in an
artificial womb constructed of the extracted uteri of women with cancer. The
scientists wrote that their study was undertaken to "... obtain the first early
human pregnancy in vitro because future complete ectogenesis should not be
ruled out."[6] More recently, Japanese scientists incubated a partially developed
goat kid from 120 days (the equivalent of the 20th to 24th gestational week of
a human fetus) until it was ready to be born 17 days later. Despite obvious
developmental problems with the resulting kid[7] the scientists were reported to
have been "pleased" with the results, making it likely that such work will
continue in the future.

2. "Severance" and "Right to Life" Abortion Theory

One of the dominant theories in moral theory on abortion is Severance theory.
Severance theorists[8] propose that abortion is moral because a woman's right
"to control her body" overrides any right a fetus might have to life.[9] What
Severance theorists assume is that the right of the mother to bodily autonomy,
and any right to life held by the fetus, are in conflict if the woman does not

want to carry the pregnancy to term. They assume, in other words, a state of medical technology not yet advanced enough to enable a woman to terminate her *pregnancy* without terminating the *life of the fetus.* If, however, it were possible for a woman to terminate her pregnancy without ending the fetus's life, Severance theorists believe this would be the only moral solution to unwanted pregnancy.

Judith Jarvis Thomson's view on this point, which utilizes her well-known violinist analogy, is typical:

> ... while I am arguing for the permissibility of abortion in some cases, I am not arguing for the right to secure the death of the unborn child.... I have argued that you are not morally required to spend nine months in bed. sustaining the life of the violinist; but to say this is by no means to say that if, when you unplug yourself, there is a miracle and he survives, you then have a right to turn round and slit his throat.[10]

Similarly, Christine Overall, who explicitly recognizes that "... in the future, expulsion from the uterus will ordinarily not result in the death of the embrvo/foetus"[11] contends that "The pregnant woman (or anyone else, e.g., a physician) has no right to kill the embryo/foetus."[12]

The manner in which severance theory justifies abortion logically compels its adherents to embrace ectogenesis as a solution to the moral difficulties they believe abortion poses. Ectogenesis enables a woman to evacuate an unwanted fetus—thereby exercising her right to bodily autonomy—without forcing her to violate any right a fetus might have to life. Thus, ectogenesis eliminates the aspect of abortion (the death of the fetus) that Severance theorists believe undesirable.

Compared to the intricacies of Severance abortion theory, the Right to Life position on abortion is simple and unambiguous. Adherents decry abortion as murder because they believe that a fetus, either as a human being or a potential human being, has a right to life. Because the termination of pregnancy has been seen as inextricable from the death of the fetus, abortion—because it causes the death of the fetus—has been seen as morally wrong.

Because ectogenetic technology would mean that abortion need no longer entail the death of the fetus[13] abortion can no longer be objected to on the ground that it violates the fetus's right to life. Thus, Right to Life theorists are logically compelled to welcome ectogenetic technology as a solution to the problematic aspects of abortion they describe.

3. Methodology

The study was conducted to investigate women's responses to ectogenesis, and whether their responses would cohere with the responses to the technology to which Severance and Right to Life abortion theorists are logically committed. It was predicted that women's construction of abortion would fundamentally differ from that articulated by Severance theorists, and that this would lead most women to reject ectogenesis as a moral solution to unwanted pregnancy. Forty-five Australian women, all resident in the state of Victoria, were interviewed in groups of between five and ten participants. Women with similar attitudes towards the morality of abortion were interviewed together. Women were recruited to the project through community and mass-media advertising.

Interview sessions lasted between one and two hours, and were recorded. Women were asked for their responses to five scenarios, of which the most important to the concerns of this paper were the "Abortion" and "Ectogenesis" scenarios, which read as follows:

"Abortion"—If pregnant with a child you could not keep, would you choose to have an abortion, or would you choose to have the child and give it up adoption? Why?

"Ectogenesis"—Imagine that you are two months pregnant. You do not want to raise the child or are unable to do so and thus must decide between having an abortion or carrying the child to term and giving it up for adoption. As you are considering these options, a doctor approaches you and tells you that you have a third option. Thanks to technology, it is now possible for you to abort your fetus without killing it. Your fetus can be extracted from your body and transferred to an artificial womb where it will be grown until it is able to live outside of that artificial womb (at around nine months) then will be put up for adoption. The doctor informs you that this procedure carries no more medical risks or inconvenience to you than the traditional abortion method.[15] Would you choose this third option?

Participants also completed a questionnaire designed to collect demographic and other bas information. Content analysis technique was used to analyze the transcribed interviews. Given the small, unrepresentative nature of the sample, standard warnings apply regarding the applicability of the findings to the population of Australian women. The names of all the women quoted in this paper are pseudonyms.

4. Women's Response to Ectogenesis

The data demonstrated a significant discrepancy between the attitudes of Severance and Right to Life theorists towards ectogenesis, and women's[15] attitudes towards the technology. An analysis of women's words reveals that the discrepancy between their attitudes and the attitudes of ethicists is grounded in the inadequate understanding both Severance and Right to Life theorists have of the framework within which women consider the morality of abortion; a framework which enables both women in favor of and women opposed to abortion rights of women to disagree on the morality of abortion, but agree on the moral unacceptability of ectogenesis.

A. Women in Favor of Abortion Rights

Women in favor of abortion rights view abortion as a moral response to unwanted pregnancy. This view is grounded in their beliefs about the moral responsibilities of mothers to their fetuses and the children they could become. Women in this group believe that a woman has a responsibility to either gestate, bear and raise her fetus and the resulting child or, if she is unable to undertake these responsibilities, to abort the fetus and so by doing prevent the further development of the fetus and the consequent creation of a child to which she has wide ranging and inescapable responsibilities. This perspective on the moral meaning and justification of abortion radically differs from that provided by Severance theorists, who justify abortion on the grounds that it enables women to exercise their right to bodily autonomy. The way women in favor of abortion rights shape the abortion dilemma makes coherent their rejection of ectogenesis.

What comes through clearly in the responses of women in favor of abortion rights is the responsibility they feel for their fetuses and the children they could become; a responsibility that seems to be derived not only from their sense of duty to a vulnerable being dependent on their care, but from the strong emotional response the fetus, as a being that could become their child, generates within them. The response of one of the participants, Charity, pictures some of these feelings:

> ... when you have an abortion, you are making a decision about your own body and about that human's life. Whereas, if you give it away, someone else is making all those decisions, or technology is making all the decisions.... I imagine that my decisions would affect my child in a more humane manner, because I've got my child's interests at heart. And that's why I'd decide to terminate, for that child's sake. If you give it away to technology, you don't know what you're doing.

Mothers, women in this group argue, may restrict their role to simply the genetic or gestational contributors to the life of their fetuses and the children they could become, but good mothers are ones that accept and perhaps even rejoice in the role of nurturer and parent of their fetus/child.[16] However, if a woman is unable to undertake the significant responsibilities entailed in being a good mother to her fetus/child, women in favor of abortion rights believe it morally acceptable—and in many cases morally laudable—for her to acquit herself of these responsibilities by choosing to terminate the life of the fetus.

Women's sense of responsibility to their fetus, as a vulnerable human for whom they had a specific duty of care, can be seen in the concern they repeatedly voiced about the fate of the fetus in the ectogenetic womb. Women worried, in other words, that once the fetus was removed from their bodies—the realm in which they exercised control over the fetus and thus could ensure its protection—it could fall prey to a wide array of physical, emotional, and social risks. For instance Emily, a woman interviewed, was concerned that a fetus reared in an ectogenetic womb wouldn't be a "proper fetus with every limb to it," while another research participant, Carey, worried about the "emotional, spiritual and mental" well-being of an artificially gestated fetus. These are just two examples amongst many that demonstrate the sense of duty women in the sample felt they had to protect their vulnerable fetus from the dangers it could encounter if removed from the protection of their bodies. Women in favor of abortion rights believed these were risks to which a good mother would not expose her fetus.

The other aspect of women's sense of responsibility to their fetuses derives not from the fetus's vulnerability and dependence upon them, but from the fetus's status as a being that could become their child. Women's belief in the power and inviolable nature of the maternal/fetus-child bond is evidenced by the concerns they express about relinquishing their fetus/child to an ectogenetic womb. This can be seen in research participant Callie's conclusions about the moral implications of "putting another person on the planet":

> No matter what you thought, there's a life here, and you are in some way responsible ... you are responsible for putting another person on the planet ... they would have to come back, or they'd be wanting their medical history.... You are still responsible for them.

If the fetus is born, women believe it will be *their* child, and they believe they have an extensive range of obligations to children that are theirs; foremost amongst them is the obligation to raise them. Over and over again women ground their rejection of adoption[17] and ectogenesis in a belief that it would be morally irresponsible of them to bring a child into the world they were unwilling or unable to parent. When Jacinta worries about not being able to "control what was happening" with a child given away, and Charity worries about damaging a child "... by not having any influence on them," both women underscore belief that women have a moral responsibility to raise their own[18] children. To bring a child into existence is to accept responsibility for their child's well-being, perhaps for life. As Carey explains, once you have put "another person on the planet," regardless of who rears them "... you are ... responsible for them."

This belief about the nature of maternal responsibility elucidates the rejection by women in this group of both adoption and ectogenesis as irresponsible abdications by women of their maternal responsibilities. This is because in both cases the child remains alive, and women believe that if their child is alive, it is their responsibility to nurture it in utero, to give birth to it, and to raise it once it is born. To abandon one's fetus to a machine constitutes a morally unacceptable abandonment of a woman's maternal duty to care for her fetus.

If a good mother raises her own children, the only solution for a woman who does not want or is unable to undertake this task is for her to prevent her child *coming into existence in the first place*. One suspects that the ideal solution for many women in this situation would be to turn back the clock to a time before they became pregnant. However, this being impossible, women are forced to embrace the only solution available to the quandary they articulate: abortion. What this suggests is that what women intend in choosing abortion is not only to terminate their *pregnancy*, but to end the *life of their fetus*. Charity sums up this position well when she says:

> ... my decision to have an abortion would be the decision I made to care for the child that was within me. So to have the child outside somewhere else would be more cruel to me than just ending it because it's giving the child no help. It's still just saying, "well, it's not my problem" ... when you have an abortion you are making a decision about your own body and about that human's life.

Although never articulated directly, women in this group clearly felt that to terminate their fetus was not necessarily to visit upon it a punishment. In other words, the fact that abortion results in the death of the fetus does not necessarily mean that women believe they wrong their fetus by aborting it. A moral abortion decision is based on the woman's caring evaluation of the outcome of continuing the pregnancy for both herself and her fetus/child as an interconnected unit.[19] The woman must evaluate the impact on herself of rearing the child and how her response to that task would consequently affect the fetus and child it could become. If the woman's decision to abort is based on her caring evaluation of the outcome of continuing the pregnancy for her maternal fetal-child unit, abortion is not only seen as permissible, but often the most moral solution in the situation. Gillian captures the nature of the interconnectedness between a woman and fetus when she says:

> I was thinking about the baby too. The adoption part was still not an issue in my decision. But I thought definitely for the baby, I didn't want it.

How much more can you think about the baby—what a miserable life it was going to have. I just didn't want it.

A number of assumptions underlie the belief of a number of women, here articulated by Gillian, that a mother's decision to abort based on an evaluation that continuing the pregnancy would harm her maternal/fetal-child unit, is morally justified. I will now seek to identify and explicate these assumptions briefly.

The first belief concerns what I have called the maternal/fetal unit. As already noted, women in this group believe that mothers and their children should remain together through the gestational period, and through the remainder of the child's dependent life. Thus in the quote above, Gillian is weighing the impact of abortion on her maternal child unit as against the impact of her raising the child. Neither adoption nor ectogenesis has a place in her considerations because they constitute in her mind a morally unacceptable abandonment of her responsibility to her fetus.

The second assumption underlying this line of reasoning is that the fetus is not the moral equivalent of a child born. Although infanticide was not a topic that arose in the majority of interviews, it is this researcher's opinion that women in this group would not view the desire of a woman to kill her *child*, because she viewed the prospects for their maternal/fetal child unit unfavorably, in the same light that they would view her decision to kill her *fetus* for the same reason. Women, in other words, view abortion as a way to *prevent the creation* of something for which, once is comes into being, they will be inescapably responsible.[20]

The third assumption underlying the words of Gillian and women who share her point of view is that the killing of one being by another is not necessarily a morally unacceptable act.[21] Predicated on their belief that the mother and her fetus/child should remain as a unit, and that the fetus does not yet have the moral significance of the child, women believe that a loving and caring assessment by the mother that her maternal/fetal child unit will be harmed were she to allow her child to be born constitutes adequate justification for a woman to choose to terminate the life of her fetus through abortion. If the woman's intentions and motives in choosing abortion are to do what is best for her maternal/fetal child unit, she can be understood to be "killing from care."[22] For women in this group, a decision to "kill from care" can often be seen to be the most responsible choice she can make to resolve an unwanted pregnancy.

Women's reasoning regarding the morality of abortion and adoption as solutions to unwanted pregnancy informs their perspective on ectogenesis. Ectogenesis results in the creation of a child to which the woman feels a maternal sense of responsibility. It creates, in other words, a woman's "own" child, and it is *precisely this event that women seek to avoid by choosing abortion*. Thus women in favor of abortion rights reject ectogenesis because it both constitutes an impermissible abandonment by the woman of her responsibility to care for her fetus, and results in her assuming maternal responsibility for a child that she is either unwilling or unable to assume.

Let us now turn to the framework within which women opposed to abortion rights consider the morality of abortion, and how that framework makes coherent their rejection of ectogenesis.

B. Women Opposed to Abortion Rights

The reasons that women opposed to abortion rights give for opposing abortion as a morally acceptable solution to unwanted pregnancy differ significantly from the reasons Right to Life theorists provide for deeming abortion an immoral response to unwanted pregnancy. For women opposed to abortion rights, the preservation of the life of the fetus is a necessary, but not a sufficient condition for a woman's response to unwanted pregnancy to be morally acceptable. Like women in favor of abortion rights, women in this group describe a good mother as one who accepts responsibility for the care of her fetus/child. For women opposed to abortion rights, however, there is no morally acceptable way for a woman to escape her responsibility to gestate and raise her fetus child once conception has taken place. Thus, for women in this group, a good mother must not only ensure the survival of all the fetuses she conceives, she must bear and raise the resulting children herself.

For women opposed to abortion rights, good women make motherhood their top priority. This can be seen in the high degree of suspicion these women evince about the motives and intentions of women seeking to terminate their pregnancies. Women who prefer their careers, their ski trips, or their holidays in Europe were constantly cited as examples of women with the sort of inadequate value systems that lead them to value the material aspects of life above their role, or potential role, as mothers, and thus choose abortion as a solution to unwanted pregnancy. A good mother values her role, or her potential role, as a mother beyond all other aspects of life, placing her children, and potential children, above her own interests, ambitions, and goals as an autonomous human being. For a good mother, in other words, there is no such thing as an *unwanted* pregnancy, only an *unexpected* one. A good mother's response to unexpected pregnancy is a willingness to make room in her life for the new arrival. Research participant Martina's discussion of her choice to keep her second child reflects this attitude:

... before I had [children] I would have said I wouldn't choose abortion... I think it's wrong, and I would have said adoption straight out as being the other alternative. But ... I've had to make that choice, with my second child, because we really couldn't afford it, but I decided to keep my second child because I just couldn't part with it ... it was something we talked about, but I just couldn't think of doing it ... there's too much bonding, it's too hard to do...

Despite the capacity of ectogenesis to preserve fetal life, it was soundly rejected by women opposed to abortion rights. Because good mothers gestate, birth, and raise their own fetuses/children, ectogenesis was seen by women in this group as an expensive alternative for women to "negate" their maternal responsibilities to their fetuses. Women in this group feared that women might attempt to utilize the ectogenetic womb to assuage their guilt about abortion, and thus were insistent that fetal evacuation be understood to constitute the same sort of maternal abandonment of responsibility for the fetus, and display the same sort of mistaken maternal values, as abortion. Grace's description of ectogenesis as a "cop-out" is a good example of this sort of reasoning:

> ... there are always people who are ready for a cop out ... and [ectogenesis] is an easy cop out ... it negates their responsibility. They've put the child in a machine for someone to rear and at the end of nine months it will be another human being ... but for that person it is just a cop out ... they can say ... I haven't had an abortion so therefore I haven't done anything wrong ... [but] there is something wrong with taking it out of you and sticking it in a machine.

Thus, women opposed to abortion rights reject abortion not only because it terminates the life of the fetus, but because they believe women should gestate and raise all the fetuses/children they conceive. This view of abortion explains why women in this group reject adoption and ectogenesis as immoral solutions to unwanted pregnancy. In fact, ectogenesis becomes, according to this view, even more problematic than adoption because evacuating a child to an ectogenetic womb means that not only is a woman rejecting her moral responsibility to *raise* her own child, but she is also rejecting her responsibility to *gestate* her own child. Thus, while for women in favor of abortion rights, ectogenesis is problematic because it preserves the life of the fetus, and with that life, a woman's maternal responsibilities, for women opposed to abortion rights, ectogenesis is a concern because it continues to enable women to avoid their responsibility to gestate, bear, and raise the children they conceive.

5. The Need and Responsibility for Change

How should ethicists respond to the disjuncture between women's moral framework on abortion and the moral framework dominating formal ethical discourse? If there is a need for change, in other words, who is it that needs to do the changing?

I would argue that there is a need for change, primarily[23] because of the irrelevance of moral theory to women's moral needs. If we accept that at least one of the goals of moral theory is to assist people to think clearly about the ethical dilemmas they face, and to make ethical decisions, then it is imperative that ethicists and the people whom they are seeking to guide—in this case women—are speaking the same language.

What this research demonstrates is that while much of the content of women's deliberations about unwanted pregnancy is unfamiliar to ethicists, the tone and tenor of these deliberations have the familiar ring of the moral. It is important that ethicists respect women's moral views on abortion and related questions, as well as attend to their content, if their contribution to the formal ethical debate on these subjects is to be meaningful.

Acknowledgement

I am indebted to Professor Peter Singer, Dr. Justin Oakley, and Ms. Lynn Gillam for their comments on previous drafts of this paper.

NOTES

1. Discussion of abortion has evolved to the point where the use of the word "baby" or "fetus," "pro-life" or "pro-choice" indicates sympathy for one or the other side of the argument. In this paper I have opted for the description of "fetus" when the life remains within the woman's body, and baby when it is outside. The terms "opposed to abortion rights" and "in favor of abortion rights" have been used for those who label themselves "pro-life" and "pro-choice" respectively. These choices were made in the admittedly futile hope of offending no one, and the more realistic one that whatever offence is caused will be evenly distributed amongst those on both sides of the controversy.

2. Viability is typically described as the potential of the fetus to be born alive, and to survive independently of its mother—albeit with artificial aid.

3. This figure is a survival rate only and does not reflect the high percentage of extremely low birth weight infants who suffer some form of physical, psychological, social, and/or intellectual disablement as a result of their extreme prematurity.

4. The usual duration of a pregnancy is 40 weeks, and typical birth weights around 3500g.

5. Dr. N. Campbell, personal communication (1991).

6. C. Bulletti et al., "Early Human Pregnancy In Vitro Utilizing an Artificially Perfused Uterus," *Fertility and Sterility* 49 (June 1988), pp. 991–996.

7. It was unable to stand or breathe by itself, a consequence of the sedatives administered to keep it from swallowing the "amniotic fluid" in its gestational sac. See Peter Hadfield, "Japanese Pioneers Raise Kid in Rubber Womb," *The New Scientist* (25 April 1992), p. 5.

8. Amongst the ranks of severance theorists are Mary Anne Warren, Judith Jarvis Thomson, Christine Overall, and Sissela Bok.

9. This point has been argued with the right to life of the fetus both accepted and rejected as a premise.

10. J. J. Thomson, "A Defence of Abortion," in *Applied Ethics*, ed. Peter Singer (Oxford: Oxford University Press, 1987), pp. 37–56.

11. C. Overall, *Ethics and Human Reproduction: A Feminist Analysis* (London: Allen and Unwin, 1987).

12. Overall, op cit.

13. In fact, our current ectogenetic capacities mean that late second and third trimester abortions need not entail the death of the fetus. That the "rescue" of the fetus via ectogenetic wombs has not been suggested by Right to Life political organizations lends credence to the argument made in this paper that the destruction of fetal life is only one of the objections Right to Lifers have to abortion.

14. It is unlikely that, were ectogenesis to become a reality, fetal evacuation would be as medically safe for women as current vacuum aspiration abortion methods. However, the scenario was shaped in this way in order to curtail certain areas of discussion.

15. For simplicity's sake, I shall refer at times to the values, beliefs, and opinions of women surveyed in this study as those of "women." Readers should bear in mind that the current sample can not be considered representative of the population of Australian women.

16. For the sake of brevity, I shall use the expression "fetus/child" in some instances as shorthand for the more cumbersome "fetus, and the child it could become."

17. The rejection of adoption by women in favor of abortion rights has been seen as one of the most interesting and controversial findings of this study. The concerns of this paper, however, restrict further discussion of this finding here.

18. The scenarios used in this research made it impossible to distinguish whether a woman felt a "fetus/child" was "her own" because of her genetic contribution, gestational contribution, or some combination of both.

19. Henceforth to be referred to as the maternal/fetal-child unit.

20. Of course, this raises questions about the precise point at which women consider the fetus to obtain moral significance, and the reasons women have for choosing this point. Unfortunately, the scope of the research precluded my further exploring the nature of women's reasoning on this point.

21. The ethical debate around euthanasia is also challenging the notion that killing—for reasons other than self-defense—is to commit a moral wrong. Of course, the fact that people at issue regarding euthanasia are both beings who have been born, and are or were at one time competent makes the relevant considerations in these cases substantially different to those pertinent when the killing of fetuses through abortion is at issue.

22. I am indebted to Dr. Michael Smith at the Philosophy Department at Monash University for coining this phrase.

23. There is another argument to be made in favor of ethicists respecting and attending to women's abortion framework; an argument that focuses primarily on the conformity of women's judgments to well-known standards for moral judgments. However, space constraints prohibit my making this argument here.

Five

OUT OF BODY GESTATION: IN WHOSE BEST INTERESTS?

Rosemarie Tong

Compared to our ancestors, we have far more control over the course of our reproductive destinies. Most of us probably know someone who uses a contraceptive, has been sterilized, has had an abortion, or is being "treated" for infertility. There is considerable debate whether infertility is best understood as a disease or a social construct. If infertility is not a disease, it cannot be treated; at most remedies can be found for it.[1] Reproductive technologies include DI (donor insemination), ICSI (intracytoplasmic sperm injection), IVF (in vitro fertilization), GIFT (gamete intrafallopian transfer), ZIFT (zygote intrafallopian transfer), ET (embryo transfer), or SET (surrogate embryo transfer),[2] is involved in negotiations for an egg donor or an embryo donor, or is looking for a woman willing to serve as a surrogate mother. It is likely that many of us have either personally used or considered using one or more of these technologies.

Our world is very different from the world a hundred years ago or even twenty-five years ago. In the past, the usual result of sexual intercourse between fertile people was pregnancy. If fertile people wished to avoid pregnancy, they had to refrain from sexual intercourse, or use a mode of birth control that was probably unreliable. Equally limited were the choices of infertile people. If they wished to have children in their lives, their main options were adoption, foster parenthood, paying special attention to their nieces and nephews, or choosing a child-centered career such as pediatrics or elementary school teaching.

Today, as a result of various technological developments, sexually active fertile people do not have to have children, and infertile people do not have to remain childless. Increasingly, people can control whether, when, and how they are going to beget and bear children. In fact, through the prenatal screening of embryos and the pre-implantation diagnosis of pre-embryos, people can largely determine what kind of child they will have. An embryo (as defined by the German Embryonic Protection Act) is a "fertilized, human egg cell, capable of development from the moment of cell union."[3] A pre-embryo (as described by the American Fertility Society) is "the entity existing before the development of the genetically distinct individual 'embryo'."[4]

It is not unusual for prospective parents to abort their genetically diseased embryos or, if they are in an in vitro fertilization program, to discard their genetically diseased pre-embryos. Some of these aborted embryos and discarded pre-embryos are afflicted with serious genetic diseases such as Tay-Sachs, but others of them are only mildly diseased, and still others are entirely healthy, their only perceived disadvantage being their sex, for example. Sex selection is any of a number of either pre- or post-implantation techniques used to prevent the birth of a particular sex infant. Clearly, we can predict that if gene therapy is ever sufficiently developed to permit the physical, intellectual, and even "moral" enhancement of one's children,[5] many prospective parents will want to use this technology to control the kind of children they procreate. Given all the developments and promised developments in reproductive technology, it is not unreasonable to envision ectogenesis—growing a human fetus to term totally outside of a woman's womb—as the culmination of reproductive technology. For as soon as we are able to control our progeny's genetic composition, we will also want to control their environment, beginning with the uterine environment. Perfect genes will demand perfect wombs, and it is precisely this demand that I wish to examine with a critical feminist lens.

This is not the first time in human history that significant attention has been paid to the possibility of ectogenesis. In fact, this is the third time since the early 1900s that ectogenesis has warranted heated debate. My intent in this essay is to discuss the technology of ectogenesis in its three major incarnations: namely, (1) its appearance at the turn of the nineteenth century in the work of physiologist-geneticist J. B. S. Haldane and his critics; (2) its re-appearance in the 1970s and 1980s in a feminist debate about the liberating as opposed to oppressive features of reproductive technology; and (3) its current appearance, as the purportedly scientifically safe and totally transparent controlled environment in which fetal life together with scientific research can supposedly thrive and progress. On the basis of discussion, I will draw some conclusions about the meaning of ectogenesis for women in particular and people in general, arguing that it is a technology to be used as the exception rather than the rule.

1. The Ectogenesis Debate in the 1920s

Not until I read Susan Squires' *Babies in Bottles: Twentieth-Century Visions of Reproductive Technology*[6] was I aware that in the early 1920s the topic of ectogenesis had been vigorously debated in England. In 1923 J. B. S. Haldane published a book under the title *Daedalus, or Science and the Future* in which he listed what he regarded as the six most important biological discoveries ever made.[7] According to Haldane, four of these inventions predated the dawn of history: namely, (1) the domestication of animals, (2) the domestication of plants, (3) the domestication of fungi for the production of alcohol, and (4) my "favorite," the gradual selection of women's face and breasts as the targets of men's attention (or, as Haldane phrases it, the change in "our idea of beauty from the steatapygous Hottentot to the modern European, from the Venus of Brassempouy to the Venus of Milo").[8] To this pre-historical list Haldane added what he viewed as two futuristic biological inventions yet to come: (5) the development of bactericides, and (6) the development of sufficient means to artificially control the process of reproduction culminating in ectogenesis: total extracorporeal gestation.

In order to understand the significance of Haldane's futuristic essay—at least it was futuristic in 1923—it is important to know something about him. Born in Oxford, England in 1892, Haldane belonged to an intellectual circle which included George Bernard Shaw, H. G. Wells, Bertrand Russell, the brothers Julian and Aldous Huxley, and D. H. Lawrence, who together led the twentieth century struggle for social and sexual emancipation. Trained in the humanities as well as in the natural sciences, Haldane became an advocate of positive eugenics, understood as breeding the best human traits to benefit future generations. To his credit and up to his death in 1964 in Bhubaneswar, India, however, Haldane remained a fierce opponent of negative eugenics, insofar as it invited involuntary sterilization laws and restrictive immigration policies crafted to purge from the gene pool so-called "unfit" types—that is, the poor, the "diseased," and the racially and ethnically dark-skinned.[9]

Of paramount significance is the fact that Haldane chose for the center-piece of *Daedalus* an imagined essay read in about the year 2073 by an undergraduate described by Haldane as "rather stupid"[10] simply because the paper he presents to his professor is by then so rudimentary. After droning on for several minutes, the student proceeds to summarize some of medicine's more glorious moments, including a crucial moment that apparently came at the midpoint of the twentieth century. Comments the student:

> It was in 1951 that Dupont and Schwarz produced the first ectogenetic child.... Dupont and Schwartz obtained a fresh ovary from a woman who was the victim of an aeroplane accident, and kept it living in their medium for five years. They obtained several eggs from it and fertilized them successfully, but the problem of the nutrition and support of the embryo was more difficult, and was only solved in the fourth year.... France was the first country to adopt ectogenesis officially, and by 1968 was producing 60,000 children annually by this method...
>
> As we know ectogenesis is now universal and in [Great Britain] less than 30 per cent of children are now born of women.... The small proportion of men and women who are selected as ancestors for the next generation are so undoubtedly superior to the average that the advance in each generation in any single respect, from the increased output of first-class music to the decreased convictions for theft, is very startling. Had it not been for ectogenesis there can be little doubt that civilization would

have collapsed within a measurable time owing to the greater fertility of the less desirable members of the population in almost all countries.[11]

Apparently Haldane envisioned ectogenesis as the technological invention that will enable the human community to control human reproduction and improve the human species without requiring anyone to be sterilized or deported. He also seemed to regard it as the development that will permit human beings to totally divorce reproduction from sexuality. At long last people would be able to indulge their sexual desires without having to pay the procreative piper for their excesses with a brood of unwanted children.

Of course, as Susan Squires points out in her book, not all of Haldane's contemporaries responded to his essay enthusiastically. Among Haldane's respondents, Squires singles out Nietzsche scholar Anthony Ludovici, author of *Lysistrata, or Woman's Future and Future Woman*;[12] sexologist Norman Haire, author of *Hymen, or the Future of Marriage*;[13] socialist physician Eden Paul, author of *Chronos, or the Future of the Family*;[14] pacifist novelist Vera Brittain, author of *Halcyon, or the Future of Monogamy*;[15] and X-ray crystallographer and molecular biologist J. D. Bernal, author of *The World, the Flesh, and the Devil: An Enquiry into the Future of the Three Enemies of the Rational Soul*.[16]

Ludovici rejected ectogenesis as the plot of body-hating feminists who saw in ectogenesis their chance to escape not only their reproductive burdens and domestic duties but also, and perhaps primarily, men themselves. Ludovici feared feminism. He forecast the coming of a sexually-oppressive feminist society in which the "periodical slaughter" of male infants is avoided only because a scientific means to limit male births to one-half of one percent of the population is discovered. Only enough men to ensure an adequate supply of sperm for breeding purposes are birthed.[17]

In contrast to Ludovici, Haire welcomed ectogenesis and its potential to emancipate women and improve the species. He envisioned total ectogenesis as simply one of the ways in which women who do not wish to gestate children and/or who are not suited to do so can be liberated from this task. Perhaps more appealing to him than the possibility of ectogenesis was the idea of some women serving other women as surrogate mothers, or even of non-human animals gestating human embryos. For Haire, what seemed most important was not whether the womb used for gestation was "natural" or "artificial" but whether the women who provided the eggs for fertilization and gestation were *genetically* fit.[18]

Less concerned about the effect of ectogenesis on women's overall social status than on women's personal psychologies, Eden Paul realized that any proposal, including his, to destroy the biological family was risky. He hoped to eliminate families based on blood ties and to substitute for them a system of "scattered homes" in which children are raised by professional parents from about the age of two upwards. Still, he remained convinced that women needed to gestate and lactate, that this nine-month-plus "period ... [of] family life is essential, both for mother and child."[19] Thus, Paul rejected ectogenesis, claiming that for at least the foreseeable future women cannot be freed from this part of "Eve's curse."[20] Apparently, Paul was not prepared to cut his very large umbilical cord to the biological family he sought to destroy.

In similar vein, but for different reasons, Vera Brittain rejected ectogenesis. She claimed that whether or not natural gestation is essential for mothers, it is somehow essential for children. Specifically, Brittain commented that:

> [The] first laboratory-grown children ... suffered as much psychologically from lack of individual parental affection or they gained physiologically through being selected from the best stock. The majority of them, indeed, though most carefully exercised, dieted and exposed to sunlight, dwindled away and died about the fifth year.[21]

Her solution to the problem of sickly "lab" children was to retain ectogenesis as an option of last resort and to develop instead ways to make "childbirth painless and pregnancy definitely pleasurable."[22] Like Paul, Brittain seemed to think that the primary motivation for ectogenesis was to help women escape from "Eve's curse." Her creative solution to the problems many women experience during and as a result of pregnancy was, however, to transform "Eve's curse" into "Eve's blessing."

Interestingly, neither Haldane nor his first four commentators—Ludovici, Haire, Eden, and Brittain—had anything against the human body. They saw in ectogenesis not a repudiation of the body, but a possible way to free the body—particularly woman's body—for more pleasure. In contrast, Bernal saw in ectogenesis the possibility of replacing puny human bodies—subject, as they are, to sensory, motor, and biological constraints—with magnificent machine bodies. Bernal imagined human beings evolving into "perfect men"—that is, completely effective, "mentally-directed mechanism[s]."[23] Comments Squires: "The perfect man ends as a brain in a beaker, having begun as a fetus in a machine uterus."[24]

2. The Ectogenesis Debate in the 1970s and 1980s

Despite the uproar the idea of ectogenesis generated in intellectual circles during the 1920s, it failed to have a significant impact on the general public. At that time neither society nor science was prepared to deal with ectogenesis, and the average person expressed little interest expressed in fundamentally altering the relationship between men and women on the one hand and parents and children on the other. Not until the 1970s and 1980s did the ectogenesis debate surface again. Once again the issues at stake were male-female relations, the relationship between sexuality and reproduction, the physical and mental health of future generations, and, perhaps most importantly, the value society in general and women in particular should attach to the human body. But this time the wider public as well as the intellectually elite seemed to have a more vested interest in these issues.

Much like Eden Paul, Shulamith Firestone wished to destroy the biological family. Yet unlike Paul, Firestone thought women could and should escape "Eve's curse." Firestone's reflections on women's reproductive role led her to develop a feminist version of historical materialism in which sex rather than class is the central concept. In much the same way that Marx argued workers' liberation requires an *economic* revolution, Firestone argued women's liberation requires a *sexual* revolution.[25] Whereas the proletariat must seize the means of *production* in order to eliminate the economic class system, women must seize control of the means of *reproduction* in order to eliminate the sexual class system. No matter how much education, legal, and political equality women achieve and no matter how many women enter public industry, Firestone insisted nothing fundamental will change for women so long as natural reproduction remains the rule and artificial or assisted reproduction the exception. Natural reproduction is neither in women's best interests nor in those of the children reproduced through it. The joy of giving birth—invoked so frequently in this society—is a patriarchal myth. In reality, childbirth is "like shitting a pumpkin."[26] Moreover, said Firestone, natural reproduction is the root of further evils, especially the vice of possessiveness that generates feelings of hostility and jealousy among human beings. Favoring one child over another on account of one of them being the product of one's own ovum or sperm is precisely what must be overcome in order to end all divisive hierarchies. All biological connections—be they genetic or gestational—must be eliminated in order to achieve equality.

Firestone was not the only feminist who claimed that gender equality requires ectogenesis and the destruction of the biological family. In her novel, *Woman on the Edge of Time*, Marge Piercy told the tale of a fictional character named Connie Ramos. Connie is a late-twentieth-century, middle-aged, lower-class Chicana with a history of what society describes as "mental illness" and "violent behavior." Connie has been trying desperately to support herself and her daughter Angelina on a pittance. One day, when she is near the point of exhaustion, Connie loses her temper and hits Angelina too hard. As a result of this one outburst, a judge declares Connie an unfit mother and takes her beloved daughter away from her. Depressed and despondent, angry and agitated, Connie is committed by her family to a mental hospital, where she is selected as a human research subject for brain-control experiments. Just when things could get no worse, Connie is transported by a woman named Luciente to a future world called Mattapoisett—a world in which women are not defined in terms of reproductive functions and in which both men and women delight in rearing children. In Mattapoisett no one is a "he" or "she"; rather, everyone is a "per" (short for *person*).[27]

Unlike Brittain who rejected ectogenesis for fear that parents would not be able to love artificially-produced children, Piercy claimed there are ways to help people love "brooder" babies as much as womb-nurtured babies. In Mattapoisett, everyone gathers around the brooder and anyone, male or female, who wishes to lactate is hormonally treated to do so. Piercy reasoned that so long as both sexes have an equal biological relationship to children, both men and women will be equally connected to their children and equally eager to participate in their upbringing.

Not all feminists in the 1970s and 1980s celebrated the possibility of ectogenesis, however. Indeed, feminists such as Mary O'Brien, Adrienne Rich, Andrea Dworkin, Margaret Atwood, Gena Corea, and Robyn Rowland saw in ectogenesis the beginnings of Bernal's "perfect man": the repudiation of the body and with it women. They reasoned that women's subordination to men is caused not by women's bodies in and of themselves but rather by men's jealousy of women's reproductive abilities and subsequent desire to seize control of female biology through scientific and technological means.[28]

According to Mary O'Brien, for example, men's jealousy of women's procreative powers is rooted in the different way men and women experience and think about bringing life into the world. Specifically, O'Brien theorized that, traditionally, a woman's "reproductive consciousness" differed from a man's in at least three ways. First, the woman experienced the process of procreation as one continuous movement taking place *within* her body, whereas the man viewed this same process as a discontinuous movement taking place *outside* of his body as soon as the act of sexual intercourse was completed. Second, the woman, not the man, necessarily performed the fundamental *labor* of reproduction: pregnancy and birthing. At most the man observed the woman performing these tasks, providing her with whatever physical and psychological help he could. Third, the woman's connection to her child was always certain—she knew, at the moment of birth, the child was flesh of her flesh. In contrast, the man's connection to the child was always uncertain; he could never be absolutely sure whether a child was in fact genetically related to him. For all he knew, the child was the biological child of some other man.[29]

In O'Brien's estimation, men's "alienated" reproductive consciousness— their sense that they have very little control over whether human life goes on and whether, in particular, their own genetic legacy lives on—helps explain why men have sought to control women's reproductive power. Reinforcing O'Brien's analysis, Adrienne Rich provided specific examples of how men, and in particular physicians, diminished women's role in reproduction. She explained that male obstetricians gradually replaced female midwives, substituting their "hands of iron" (obstetrical forceps) for midwives' hands of flesh (female hands sensitive to female anatomy).[30] Male experts told women how to act during pregnancy—when to eat, sleep, exercise, have sex, and the like. In some instances, they even dictated to women how to *feel* during the process of childbirth—when to feel pain and when to feel pleasure. The overall effect of men's intrusion into the birthing process was to confuse women, since men's "rules" for women's pregnancies often clashed with women's "intuitions" about what was best for their bodies, psyches, and babies. For example, when a woman and physician disagreed about whether she needed a C-section to deliver her baby, a woman did not know whether to trust the *authority* of her physician or the *experience*, the sensations, of her own body. To the degree women were deprived of control over their pregnancies, said Rich, women started to experience pregnancy as merely an event, as something that simply happened *to* them.

Rich's analysis about the ways in which patriarchal authorities used medical science to control women's reproductive powers were further echoed in the works of yet other 1970s and 1980s feminists. Andrea Dworkin claimed that in recent years infertility experts have joined gynecologists and obstetricians to seize control of women's reproductive powers. In her estimation, the technologies of assisted reproduction are gradually making woman's reproductive consciousness just as alienated as men's.[31] With the introduction of in vitro fertilization, egg donors, and the use of surrogate mothers, a woman's experience of bringing a child into the world becomes as discontinuous as that of the man. Absent DNA analysis, a woman can be no more certain than her partner that the child born to them is indeed *their* genetic child. For all they know, the embryo transplanted into her womb is not their embryo but the embryo of some other couple. Moreover, even if a woman is certain that an embryo is related to her genetically, if she is unable or unwilling to gestate it, she may feel somewhat disconnected from it, less than its "real" mother. Dworkin speculated that were scientists to develop an artificial womb, women would lose their social status as mothers, their primary source of "leverage" in most societies, but particularly in patriarchal ones.

Agreeing with Dworkin that the new reproductive technologies might decrease women's social value, Robyn Rowland, another feminist, imagined a worst-case scenario for women: a masculinist world in which only a few superovulating women are permitted to exist, a world in which eggs are taken from women, frozen, and inseminated in vitro for transfer into artificial wombs. The replacement of women's childbearing capacity by male-controlled technology would, she claimed, leave women entirely vulnerable. She asked "what role is envisioned for women" in a world where women's "last power" is taken and controlled by men?"[32]

Clearly, in the voices of O'Brien, Rich, Dworkin, and Rowland, we hear counter versions of Ludovici's concerns. He feared feminists would use ectogenesis to make men obsolete. Only a few sperm donors would be spared extinction. In contrast, many 1970s and 1980s feminists worried just the opposite. They feared ectogenesis would lead to women's obsolescence.

3. The Ectogenesis Debate Today

As in the 1920s, the 1970s and early 1980s the ectogenesis debate lost steam. As it turned out, most people did not think either that pregnancy was an impediment to gender equality or that assisted reproduction was a masculinist plot hatched by men to seize from women their life-giving powers. For the most part, the majority of the population—feminists as well as traditionalists— agreed with Rich that women could "have their cake and eat it too." Women, they believed, could gain control of artificial as well as natural reproduction to serve women's as well as society's best interests.

Perhaps the most important reason why the ectogenesis debate failed both in the 1970s and 1980s as well as the 1920s and 1930s was that the scientific community as well as the general public believed that ectogenesis was more science fiction than science fact. Still, there were significant dissenters from this common wisdom. In 1985, Peter Singer, a philosopher, and Deane Wells, a member of the Australian Parliament, wrote a book entitled *Making Babies: The New Science and Ethics of Conception* in which they argued that ectogenesis was on the "fast track" for at least two reasons.[33]

First, fetal viability was shifting to ever earlier times due to developments in the Neonatal Intensive Care Unit (NICU). By the late 1980s it was possible to save babies born as early as six or even five and a half months, and weighing less than 100 grams.[34] Singer and Wells reasoned that before long someone would invent an incubator able to sustain a five-or even a four-and-a-half-month old fetus. Although this incubator has yet to be designed for human babies, in the 1990s some Japanese researchers incubated a partially developed goat kid from 120 days (the equivalent of the 20th to 24th gestational week of a human fetus) until birth seventeen days later. Despite serious developmental problems with the resulting kid—it was unable to stand or breathe by itself— the researchers pronounced their experiment a near success.[35]

Singer and Wells' second source of optimism about the development of ectogenesis drew inspiration from the opposite end of pregnancy—that is, from the moment of conception rather than of birth. They pointed to the then relatively new procedure of in vitro fertilization (IVF). In IVF a number of eggs are removed from a woman's ovaries and fertilized with sperm outside her body. When the fertilized eggs or zygotes are developed to about the eight cell stage, they are transferred back into either her uterus or the uterus of another woman. Although no human embryo transfer attempted more than three days after fertilization (the 32 cell stage) has implanted successfully in a woman's womb, some scientists have reportedly kept human embryos alive in

vitro for up to nine days.[36] Moreover, the fact that the fact that the United
Kingdom, for example, currently forbids experimentation on human fetuses in
vitro after fourteen days suggests that it is indeed possible to keep pre-embryos
alive for at least two weeks and maybe longer.[37]

In an attempt to decide whether the overall benefits of ectogenesis exceed
its overall harms, Singer and Wells discussed five pro-ectogenesis arguments
and five anti-ectogenesis arguments. They claimed that there are two particularly strong arguments in favor of ectogenesis. The first of these arguments
is that ectogenesis offers "an alternative to surrogate motherhood for women
who are incapable of pregnancy or for whom pregnancy is not recommended
on medical grounds."[38] Rather than contracting a surrogate mother to gestate
her and her partner's embryo, a woman who has eggs but is unable to gestate
them could instead use an artificial womb to bring the embryo to term.
Supposedly, it would be advisable for her to exercise this option in order to
avoid situations such as the one that arose in the Whitehead/Stern controversy
over Baby M,[39] in which Mary Beth Whitehead, the surrogate mother, refused
to give the Sterns, the couple who had contracted her services, the baby she
had agreed to gestate for them. An emotionally and financially exhausting
legal battle ensued. After many harrowing months, the New Jersey Supreme
Court ruled that surrogacy contracts were against the public interest. However,
the same court also ruled that it was in the best interest of the child, who was
by then two years old, to remain in the custody of the Sterns.[40] In Singer and
Wells's estimation, had an artificial womb been available, both the Sterns and
the Whiteheads could have been spared much grief.

In Singer and Wells's estimation, the second strong argument in favor of
ectogenesis is its potential to resolve the abortion controversy. Presently, there
is no way to remove a first-trimester or early second-trimester fetus from a
woman's body without killing the fetus. But subsequent to the development of
an artificial womb, a fetus could be extracted from a woman's body for
transfer and further development in it. Singer and Wells claimed that although
women have a right to be "rid of the fetus," they do not necessarily also have a
right to kill it.[41]

Having summarized what they regarded as the two strongest arguments in
favor of ectogenesis, Singer and Wells then considered what they regarded as
two more debatable arguments in favor of it. First, biological pregnancy is not
in women's best interests because, as Firestone had argued in the 1970s, the
pregnancy experience contributes to women's powerlessness outside the
domestic sphere. Second, biological pregnancy is not in children's interests
because it causes mothers to cling to their children as their lifetime special
possessions.[42] According to Singer and Wells, these arguments are weak
because there is presently no way to calculate the effects of ectogenesis on
women's and children's best interests. For all we know, ectogenesis may be
worse for women and children than biological pregnancy.

Finally, Singer and Wells addressed the possibility of using ectogenesis to keep embryos alive as a source of tissues and organs for more mature humans. They described this type of ectogenesis as "partial" as opposed to "complete" ectogenesis since its aim is not the survival of the embryo as a person but the welfare of other persons.[43] They also emphasized that for individuals who do not believe that embryos become persons until the point of viability or even later, it may indeed make sense to use embryos to save the lives of human beings whose personhood has been firmly established.

Among the anti-ectogenesis arguments Singer and Wells outlined were the following. First, they considered the same concerns about the health of "ectobabies" that Vera Brittain had raised in the 1920s ectogenesis debate. They stressed that critics are right to insist that every effort be made to protect ectobabies from serious physical and/or psychological harms. Ectogenesis must not go forward until researchers are confident that they will do no, or at least, very little, harm to future generations.[44]

In addition to this strong argument against ectogenesis, Singer and Wells presented what they regarded as three weaker arguments against it. First, ectogenesis is part of a masculinist conspiracy to rob women of their reproductive powers.[45] Second, it is an "unnatural" technology that violates God's laws.[46] Third, it is the development that will destroy our democracy, substituting for it a *Brave New World* in which state authorities selectively breed only those types of individuals likely to be maximally useful to society.[47] Singer and Wells dismissed all these arguments as unfounded. They argued that women no less than men want to use reproductive technology; that ectogenesis is no more "unnatural" than most medical technologies; and that the State has no interest in using an excessively costly technology to breed certain types of workers. Finally, Singer and Wells considered the anti-ectogenesis argument that, far from it being good to grow embryos for spare organs and extra tissue, it is murder pure and simple to do so. In this connection, they noted that for many people, personhood, together with the right to life, begins at the moment of conception.[48]

Reflecting back on the arguments both for and against ectogenesis, Singer and Wells concluded that the arguments against *complete* ectogenesis—the kind of ectogenesis intended to result in the birth of a baby—are simply not strong enough to cancel out the good that complete ectogenesis promises. No longer will surrogate mothers and contracting couples be at odds and no longer will pro-life and pro-choice forces be at war. However, added Singer and Wells, there are arguments against *partial* ectogenesis over and beyond the argument that it constitutes murder—arguments that are powerful enough to put a halt to using ectogenesis to create an organ and tissue farm. Such a use of ectogenesis threatens to erode the kindly feelings adults usually manifest toward vulnerable infants. Singer and Wells stressed that among normal humans, the sight of a newborn baby evokes feelings of protectiveness and caring, while the sight of an embryo (presumably in a jar or a photograph) does not. They then hypothesized that it might become too easy for humans to become dependent on the benefits of partial ectogenesis, which would eventually lead to a shift in adults' attitude toward children, from viewing children as unique persons to love to viewing children as resources to exploit.[49] For this reason, Singer and Wells concluded that partial ectogenesis should be rejected. Its harms overwhelm its benefits.

Although Singer and Wells established to their satisfaction that *complete* (as opposed to *partial*) ectogenesis is a morally permissible technology, their critics remained unconvinced. In particular, philosopher David James argued that even if ectogenesis provides a way to better handle surrogacy arrangements than "renting" a living woman's womb, society should not spend limited resources developing such a costly technology for a limited number of people.[50] But even though I, like James, think that we need to reconsider our health care priorities so as to secure "greater bang for our buck," if access to ectogenesis is the only way a couple can have a baby that is genetically related to them, I very much doubt that ectogenesis can or should be legally prohibited.[51] In the past, I minimized the genetic connection because our legal system has tended to value genetic parenthood over gestational parenthood in ways that have tended to privileged the father's over the mother's control of a child. But, even though this is true, I have gradually been persuaded that many women value the genetic connection just as much as men do. Women, no less than men, like to see themselves reflected in their children. At the very least, many women explain some of their children's physical and psychological weaknesses and strengths in terms of their own.

For this reason, and because of serious concerns I have about one woman using another woman's body to make a baby for her for money, I am prepared to accept the better surrogacy argument in favor of ectogenesis. However, I am not prepared to accept Singer and Wells's "abortion reconciliation" argument in favor of ectogenesis. According to Singer and Wells, women's right to an abortion is simply the right to have one's fetus extracted from one's body, and not also the right to have the fetus killed.[52] Among others, feminist philosopher Christine Overall disagrees with this interpretation of the abortion right. For Overall, abortion is primarily about the right *not to procreate*, and it is precisely this purported right that adds to the moral weight of the abortion controversy. When a woman seeks an abortion, she probably has fetal extinction and not merely fetal extraction as her goal. She simply does not want to procreate—to bring another life into the world—at that time or perhaps at any time.[53]

Overall presents and evaluates four arguments to support the view that fetal extinction rather than fetal extraction is the ultimate aim of abortion. She claims that the first argument in favor of using abortion to kill the fetus is that keeping a fetus alive against the wishes of its biological mother violates that woman's reproductive autonomy. Overall notes that although it is easy enough to free a biological mother from her social obligations to her fetus, it is not also possible to free her from her genetic and/or gestational connections to it. Since some biological mothers view abortion as a way to erase *all* their connections to the fetuses, Overall observes that anything less than the death of their fetus would fail to satisfy them.[54]

The second argument in favor of killing the fetus in Overall's estimation is that "saving the fetus against the mother's will would be like compelling her to donate organs, blood, or gametes against her will."[55] Although Overall believes that unlike organs, blood, or gametes, fetuses have a life of their own, she remains adamantly opposed to efforts aimed at "rescuing" fetuses intended for an abortion. As she sees it, it is up to the pregnant woman to decide whether, when, and how to remove the fetus from her body. She claims that forcing a woman to submit to whatever abortion procedure is most likely to preserve the life of a fetus is "comparable to a compulsory organ 'donation' in which the patient chooses organ removal but does not agree to the subsequent salvaging and use of the organ."[56]

The third argument in favor of killing the fetus, says Overall, is that "by virtue of her physical relationship to it, the biological mother is the most appropriate person—perhaps the only one—to decide the disposition of the fetus."[57] Overall supports this argument completely, insofar as not-yet-born fetuses are concerned, but only partially, insofar as born fetuses are concerned, including fetuses who survive the abortion procedure. To the extent that these latter fetuses are like premature infants, she believes their biological mothers have an obligation to take their interests, including their interests in living and being adopted, into account.

Overall's final argument in favor of killing the fetus is that "deliberately withholding the determination of the disposition of the fetus from the biological mother is yet another example of the takeover of reproduction from women."[58] In this connection philosopher Anne Donchin writes that

> ... if extrauterine gestation were to become an established practice, would not many women be pressured to adopt it—"for the good of their baby?" For within the prevailing social framework, once the practice was established, it is unlikely that only intentionally aborted fetuses would be nourished in laboratories. Any other fetus considered "at risk" for any reason would count as a potential beneficiary of laboratory observation and intervention.[59]

I think Donchin's observation is plausible. Ectogenesis would, in the minds of many, be the perfect solution to the so-called maternal-fetal conflict problem.[60] Rather than seeking to designate crack-cocaine abusing pregnant women as fetal abusers and neglectors, for example, prosecutors would instead seek court orders to remove from the wombs of these wayward mothers their fetuses. Eventually, only women with "safe" uteri would be permitted to gestate their children. At the very least, one can—as Donchin does—imagine concerned women requesting physicians to transfer their fetus from them into a safer, albeit more artificial environment.

For those who view such speculations as fanciful, consider science reporter Sharon Begley's article in which she points out that "[s]cientists now think that conditions during gestation, ranging from the torrent of hormones that flow from Mom to how well the placenta delivers nutrients to the tiny limbs and organs, shape the health of the adult that fetus becomes."[61] Moreover, continues Begley, these same scientists are convinced that so-called fetal programming best explains "adult illnesses long blamed on years of living dangerously (like dining on pizza and cupcakes)."[62] In particular, low birth weight is, cross-culturally, a predictor of a host of serious adult-onset diseases.[63]

Begley notes that "fetal programming" has been the subject of two recent National Institutes of Health conferences, both of which sought to establish connections between a variety of diseases and the conditions present in the womb during fetal gestation. In addition, she points to growing evidence that individuals who have asymmetrical features such as ears, fingers, and feet also have lower IQs. Like low birth weight, asymmetrical features may be markers, or indicators, of stress which took place during pregnancy. One conclusion of this research is that whatever stress led to the asymmetrical features could also have effects on the nervous system, causing impairments in the senses, memory, and cognition. Other studies indicate that the genes that affect the so-called stress response may become "turned off" if a fetus is exposed to stress hormones (within the womb). Thereby, the growing child may be impaired in his or her ability to handle stress in adulthood. In the words of Dr. Peter Nathanielsz, "The script written on the genes is altered by ... the environment in the womb."[64]

Perhaps the most significant feature of Begley's article is its conclusion. There Begley recollects the chapter in Huxley's *Brave New World* wherein he "describes how workers at the Central London Hatchery, where fetuses grow in special broths, adjust the ingredients of the amniotic soup depending on which kind of child they need. Children destined to work in chemical factories are treated so they can tolerate lead and calcium; those destined to pilot rockets are constantly rotated so that they learn to enjoy being upside-down."[65] Pondering this vision, Begley writes, "The quest for the secrets of fetal programming won't yield up such simple recipes. But it is already showing that the seeds of health are planted even before you draw your first breath, and that the nine short months of life in the womb shape your health as long as you live."[66]

Begley's article, I admit, caused me to ask myself whether the causes of my sons' present woes are rooted in the troubled uterine environment with which I provided them. Would, I wonder, they be healthier had they been born in an artificial womb? Perhaps. But would I feel as "bonded" to them as I feel today had they not once been part of me? Perhaps, but then again perhaps not. To be sure, as a feminist, I realize that neither genetic nor gestational connections are necessary for parenthood. I also realize that such biological connections can spawn considerable evils—the feelings of possessiveness that Firestone feared. I also know that pregnancy has kept many women in bondage and that it can be harrowing. But, having said all of this, I confess that I loved the physicality, the materiality, the emotionality of pregnancy. I cannot help but agreeing with Adrienne Rich when she writes "that female biology—the diffuse, intense sensuality radiating out from clitoris, breasts, uterus, vagina; the lunar *cycles* of menstruation; the gestation and fruition of life which can take place in the female body—has far more radical implications than we have come to appreciate,"[67] and when she proclaims that "[i]n order to live a fully human life we require not only *control* of our bodies (though control is a prerequisite) we must touch the unity and resonance of our physicality, our bond with the natural order, the corporeal ground of our intelligence."[68]

As I see it, it would be good to develop some form of artificial womb to sustain premature babies, provided they can grow in a healthy manner there. But I do not affirm substituting artificial wombs for women's wombs on a regular and routine basis. To recommend such a substitution spells the repudiation of the body, and with it everything, at least in Western culture, associated with the body, including woman herself.

Although I have certain disagreements with philosopher Leon Kass, including his conservative views on homosexual and lesbian sexual practices and parenthood, I nonetheless agree with him that it is important to celebrate our bodies equally with our minds, as co-constitutive of our humanity and as the source of our enviable diversity, our unique colors, smells, smells, sounds, textures, and tastes. Comments Kass:

> Crucial to the development of genuine sociability and culture is the perception of one's place in the line of generations. Those who aspire to autonomy and self-sufficiency are prone to forget—indeed eager to forget—that the world did not and does not begin with them. Civilization is altogether a monument to ancestors biological and cultural, to those who came before, in whose debt one always lives, like it or not. We can pay this debt, if at all, only by our transmission of life and teachings to those who come after. Mind, freely wandering, in speculation or fantasy, can forget time and relation, but a mind that thinks on the body will be less likely to do so. In the navel are one's forebears, in the genitalia our descendants. These reminders of perishability are also reminders of per-

petuation; if we understand their meaning, we are even able to transform the necessary and shameful into the free and noble. ... Embodiment is a curse only for those who believe they deserve to be gods.[69]

Babies born through ectogenesis will have genitalia, but they will not have navels; and, although I ordinarily eschew people who fixate on their navels, I have given mine recent attention, feeling somehow especially connected to my deceased mother and through her to all the human beings that have preceded me.

My hope is that in the 2000s, as in the 1920s, and then again in the 1970s and 1980s, ectogenesis will fade into the margins of human consciousness, a technology to use perhaps as the exception but not as the rule. If we view the navel as a symbol of a lifeline linked to the past, as a reminder of our need for human connection and as the stamp of our embodiment, I think we will be able to presume our humanity for another century or so. Otherwise I fear we may end up as "brains in beakers," utterly alone in our thoughts and profoundly disconnected from each other and any possible value and meaning we might have.

NOTES

1. See Patricia A. Stephenson with Marsden G. Wagner, "World Health Organization Report on the Place of In Vitro Fertilization in Infertility Care," in *Encyclopedia of Reproductive Technologies*, ed. Annette Burfoot (Boulder, Col.: Westview Press, 1999), pp. 283–288.

2. See Burfoot, *Encyclopedia of Reproductive Technologies*, pp. xi–xvii.

3. See Anne Waldschmidt, "Legislation—Germany," in Burfoot, *Encyclopedia of Reproductive Technologies*, pp. 325–326.

4. See Patricia Spallone, "Embryo Research," in Burfoot, *Encyclopedia of Reproductive Technologies*, p. 344.

5. LeRoy Walters and Julie Gage Palmer, *The Ethics of Human Germ Therapy* (New York: Oxford University Press, 1997), pp. 99–142.

6. Susan Squires, *Babies in Bottles: Twentieth-Century Visions of Reproductive Technology* (New Brunswick, NJ: Rutgers University Press, 1994).

7. J. B. S. Haldane, *Daedalus, or Science and the Future*, in *Haldane's Daedalus Revisited*, ed. Krishna R. Dronamraju (Oxford: Oxford University Press, 1995), pp. 23–50.

8. *Ibid.*, p. 35.

9. Krishna R. Dronamraju, "Introduction," in Dronamraju, *Haldane's Daedalus Revisited*, p. 14.

10. Haldane, *Daedalus, or Science and the Future*, p. 14.

11. *Ibid.*, p. 42.

12. Anthony M. Ludovici, *Lysistratra, or Woman's Future and Future Woman* (London: Kegan Paul, Trench, and Trubner, 1927).

13. Norman Haire, *Hymen, or the Future of Marriage* (London: Kegan Paul, Trench, and Trubner, 1927).

14. Eden Paul, *Chronos, or the Future of the Family* (London: Kegan Paul, Trench, and Trubner, 1930).

15. Vera Brittain, *Halycyon, or the Future of Monogamy* (London: Kegan Paul, Trench, and Trubner, 1929).

16. J. D. Bernal, *The World, the Flesh, and the Devil: An Enquiry into the Future of the Three Enemies of the Rational Soul* (London: Kegan Paul, Trench, and Trubner, 1930).

17. Ludovici, *Lysistrata, or Woman's Future and Future Woman*, p. 95.

18. Haire, *Hymen, or the Future of Marriage*, pp. 87–88.

19. Paul, *Chronos, or the Future of Marriage*, p. 34.

20. *Ibid.*

21. Brittain, *Halycyon, or the Future of Monogamy*, p. 77.

22. *Ibid.*

23. Bernal, *The World, the Flesh, and the Devil*, p. 46.

24. Squires, *Babies in Bottles*, p. 88.

25. Shulamith Firestone, *The Dialectic of Sex* (New York: Bantam Books, 1970).

26. Ibid.

27. Marge Piercy, *Woman on the Edge of Time* (New York: Fawcett Crest Books, 1976).

28. Adrienne Rich, *Of Woman Born* (New York: W. W. Norton, 1979), p. 11.

29. Mary O'Brien, *The Politics of Reproduction* (Boston: Routledge and Kegan Paul, 1981), pp. 35–36.

30. Rich, *Of Woman Born*, p. 111.

31. Andrea Dworkin, *Right-wing Women* (New York: Coward-McCann, 1983), pp. 187–188.

32. Robyn Rowland, "Reproductive Technologies: The Final Solution to the Woman Question" in *Test-tube Women*, ed. Ruth Arditti, Rebecca Klein, and Shelley Minden (London: Pandora Press, 1984), p. 45.

33. Peter Singer and Deane Wells, *Making Babies: The New Science and Ethics of Conception* (New York: Charles Scribner's Sons, 1985), pp. 117–118 [this volume, pp. 10–11].

34. Ibid.

35. P. Hadfield, "Japanese Pioneers Raise Kid in Rubber Womb," *The New Scientist* (25 April 1992), p. 5.

36. Singer and Wells, *Making Babies*, p. 117.

37. John A. Robertson, "Embryo Research," University of Western Ontario Law Review 24 (1986): 15–37.

38. Singer and Wells, *Making Babies*, p. 118.

39. Phyllis Chesler, *The Sacred Bond: The Legacy of Baby M* (New York: Time Books, 1988).

40. "Excerpts from Decision by New Jersey Supreme Court in the Baby M Case," *New York Times* (4 February 1988), p. B6.

41. Singer and Wells, *Making Babies*, p. 120 [this volume, p. 12].

42. Ibid, pp. 120–122 [this volume, pp. 12–14].

43. Ibid, p. 123–124 [this volume, pp. 15–16].

44. Ibid, pp. 124 [this volume, p. 16].

45. Ibid, pp. 124–125 [this volume, pp. 16–17].

46. Ibid, p. 125–126 [this volume, pp. 17–180].

47. Ibid, p. 126 [this volume, p. 18].

48. Ibid. [this volume, p. 18].

49. Ibid, pp. 132–133 [this volume, pp. 23–25].

50. David N. James, "Ectogenesis: A Reply to Singer and Wells," *Bioethics* 1 (1987), pp. 90–95.

51. John A. Robertson, *Children of Choice* (Princeton, N.J.: Princeton University Press, 1994), pp. 22–44.

52. Singer and Wells, *Making Babies*, p. 132.

53. Christine Overall, *Human Reproduction: Principles, Practices, Policies* (Toronto: Oxford University Press, 1993) p. 67.

54. Ibid. See also Leslie Cannold, "Women, Ectogenesis, and Ethical Theory," in this volume.

55. Ibid, p. 69.

56. Ibid.

57. Ibid.

58. Ibid.

59. Anne Donchin, "The Growing Feminist Debate Over the New Reproductive Technologies," *Hypatia* 4 (1989), p. 144.

60. John A. Robertson, "Procreative Liberty and the Control of Conception, Pregnancy, and Childbirth," *Virginia Law Review* 69 (1983), pp. 405–464.

61. Sharon Begley, "Shaped by Life in the Womb," *Newsweek* 134 (9 September 1999), p. 51.

62. Ibid.

63. Ibid, p. 52.

64. Ibid, p. 57.

65. Ibid.

66. Ibid.

67. Rich, *Of Woman Born*, p. 17.

68. Ibid.

69. Leon R. Kass, *Toward a More Natural Science: Biology and Human Affairs* (New York: Free Press, 1985), p. 291.

Six

WHAT'S SO GOOD ABOUT NATURAL MOTHERHOOD? (IN PRAISE OF UNNATURAL GESTATION)

Gregory Pence

1. Introduction

For over thirty years, medical researchers have been trying to develop an artificial womb. Gestation a baby this way is technically called *ectogenesis.* Some recent research shows promise by creating scaffolds of biodegradable material molded into the shape of the interior of a human uterus, to which embryos (left over from in vitro fertilization) were added. Professor Hung-Ching Liu of Cornell University's Center for Reproductive Medicine and Fertility nurtured the embryos with hormones and nutrients and they attached to the artificial uterine wall and grew for six days, until the experiment was halted. Professor Yoshinori Kuwabara has been doing similar research in Japan with goat fetuses in artificial tanks filled with amniotic fluids.

Should this kind of research find success, premature babies might be viable who now are not. In addition, as the artificial womb is perfected, it might become an alternative to traditional gestation.

Currently, "ECMO" (Extra Corporeal Membrane Oxygenation) functions as an artificial lung for premature babies with inadequate lung development. In function, it resembles the bypass machines used in heart transplantation. After entubating a large vein in the baby's neck, blood flows by gravity through a plastic bladder, where a membrane oxygenator also removes carbon dioxide, after which the oxygenated blood is warmed and returned to the body through an artery in the neck. This machine is now common in all neonatal intensive care units (NICUs) and this development shows that ectogenesis may not be as far off as commonly thought.

Futurists frequently say we need to think through possible technological breakthroughs before they are implemented, so that we can assess their impact in advance. This essay is a first step in that direction, but with a twist. Almost always, what such futurists mean is that we should stop such breakthroughs until we are certain that all their consequences are benign. In this essay, I argue that the onus of proof, after primate studies showed such wombs safe, should be on critics who would deny their use, especially as potentially therapeutic last-ditch efforts for dying, premature babies.

2. The Emotional Symbolism of the Artificial Womb

Like human cloning, the artificial womb has powerful symbolic connotations. To some it would be the essence of a *Blade Runner* future, with babies gestated inside cold, inhumane machines lacking a natural mother's concern and bodily comfort. To such critics, babies raised in such an alien environment would inevitably be psychologically traumatized. So powerful is the symbolism of the artificial womb that to them, rather than a human good, it would actually be a worst-case scenario of the future of reproductive medicine.

Motherhood also symbolizes all that is comforting and safe and personal, the opposite of what is dangerous, foreign, state-controlled, and harmful. If ontogeny repeats phylogeny in the history of ethics, our most ancient ethics will be about our primordial roles, as son, as mother or father, as teacher, as craftsman, and so on. For this reason, changes in gestation may seem especially dangerous to conventional notions of family and female nurturing. Extracorporeal gestation can attack a very primordial world-view about what humans are and their world. If I see a young woman with two small children, my first thought is of her as the woman who gestated and is raising those children. That may be incorrect, but odds are that it is true. With extracorporeal gestation, a man could much more easily be the primary nurturer and we would not know if the baby had been gestated by a woman or ectogenesis.

With such assumptions about motherhood in place, and because we have been conditioned by science fiction and alarmists to feel this way, a massive "yuk" reaction can be predicted about any progress towards an artificial womb. Indeed, that is almost certainly inevitable. For many people, such news would be an emotional kick-in-the-stomach, a frightening threat to their sense of normalcy. As such, medicine will need to introduce the artificial womb carefully in clearly justified cases, such as those discussed at the end of this piece.

Recently, some bioethicists knowledgeable about neurobiology, cognitive science, and evolutionary biology have embraced trends in these fields to integrate current ideas with inferences about what practices in human evolution were advantageous adaptations. So certain kinds of cooperative behavior, unforced choices, and self-interested seeking have been argued to have been selected for in evolution.

Unfortunately, authors who argue this way usually commit (what I call) the *Evolved Implies Ought Fallacy*, which states that because human evolution to date involved practice X, therefore, practice X is moral. The fallacy of this line of thinking is immediately obvious when one considers that the genes of many past humans were spread by rape after conquest of a village, incest, or forced sex with slaves. Alexander the Great left men behind in cities he conquered in a deliberate policy of miscegenation. And by the time he did this, two thousand years ago, humans had already evolved into the basic form we know today. Who knows what terrible behaviors were necessary for evolution in the millions of years before Alexander? These considerations forestall the argument that natural gestation is morally obligatory because humans evolved this way. If and when it becomes practical and safe to gestate in an artificial womb, appealing to evolution will not be relevant.

We also have many beliefs and intuitions about motherhood that affect the emotional reaction to the idea of the artificial womb. Perhaps none of them are true. For example, beliefs about a by-gone golden era of ideal motherhood may be false. Social historian Stephanie Coontz's *The Way We Never Were* describes a very different view of motherhood in the American past:

> ... the middle-class Victorian family depended for its existence on the multiplication of other families who were too poor and powerless to retreat into their own little oases and who therefore had to provision the oases of others. ... For every nineteenth-century middle-class family that protected its wife and child within the family circle, then, there was an Irish or a German girl scrubbing the floors in that middle-class home, a Welsh boy mining coal to keep the home-baked goodies warm, a black girl doing the family laundry, a black mother and child picking cotton to be made into clothes for the family, and Jewish or an Italian daughter in a sweatshop making "ladies" dresses or artificial flowers for the family to purchase.[1]

The meaning of motherhood has undergone much transformation. There are certainly many meanings of the word "mother," so which is the essential one in "natural motherhood"? Is it the egg donor? Embryo source? Female genetic ancestor? The mitochondrial DNA donor (in egg of cloned embryo)? The gestator or surrogate mother? The woman who actually adopts and raises the child? The person who is the most important to the child emotionally, the nurturer (who could be the dad or aunt or teacher)?

Although there are many confusing and conflicting meanings of motherhood, for our purposes here we will assume that a woman gestating a fetus created from her own egg and a man's sperm, which combined sexually for form an embryo, is a "natural mother." It is this sense of natural motherhood that some would see as under attack with a successful, safe artificial womb.

3. A Brief History of Assisted Reproduction

Every issue in bioethics has a pedigree. Without understanding that pedigree, we wander in the dark of history, not knowing where we are. The history of reproductive ethics is especially important to understand because reproductive ethics is a very personal topic for most people.

The artificial womb is the ultimate form of assisted reproduction. Within the history of reproductive ethics, the history of the ethics of assisted repro-

duction is especially germane to thinking about the ethics of the artificial
womb. So a brief overview of past ethical issues about assisted reproduction
'l guide us in thinking about the future.

Most writing about assisted reproduction portrays it as an attack on the
ional family. A centuries-old anti-intellectual tradition in Western culture
ways attacked any change related to sex or motherhood. Every innovation in reproductive ethics has been met with criticism and resistance by the
status quo.

Perhaps the most famous example is anesthesia in childbirth. For millions
of years, women had to birth their babies in pain. Julius Caesar is said by
legend to have been born by the childbirth operation bearing his name, but in
any case, it saved the lives of many babies and mothers. Similarly, anesthesia,
first discovered by Georgia primary care physician Crawford Long and later
re-discovered by a Boston dentist, changed the birthing process for millions of
women. When first practiced, anesthesia during childbirth was denounced from
the pulpits because of the verse, practically at the start of the Bible in Genesis,
where God says to Eve (after her sin of tempting Adam in the Garden of
Eden), "I will greatly multiply thy sorrow and thy conception; in sorrow thou
shalt bring forth children; and thy desire shall be to thy husband, and he shall
rule over thee." (Genesis 3:16)

Artificial insemination of husband's (AIH) sperm into his wife was used
by physician J. Marion Sims to produce a pregnancy in the late 1860s but the
baby miscarried and Sims was denounced as a pervert, as was a Brooklyn
physician Robert Latou Dickenson in the 1890s. Not until the 1960s did
medicine and society tolerate AIH, so a century of infertile couples were
denied babies in America because of intellectual rigidity.

In vitro fertilization created a storm of controversy in the early 1970s.
Baby Louise Brown was only born after hundreds of embryos and fetuses
miscarried. Nevertheless, today hundreds of thousands of babies exist worldwide, not as bought commodities, but as some of the most-cherished babies
ever conceived.

As I will discuss below, so-called "surrogate mothers" or surrogates
created controversy in the 1980's, especially when the mothers were paid, as in
the case of Baby M in New Jersey, which had to go to the New Jersey Supreme
Court for final disposition. Initially, people had a strong "yuk" response to
commercial surrogacy, dubbing such women "rent-a-wombs," but gradually
this response has faded as people understood that women who undertook this
task for another woman were not mindless slaves entrapped by the offer of
money nor shameless renters of their wombs. And altruistic surrogacy without
the exchange of money enjoys the approval now of many Americans.

As reproductive technology has rapidly progressed, each new controversy
emits cries that the sky is falling, whether it be egg donation, intracytoplasmic
sperm injection (ICSI), embryo selection against lethal genetic diseases,

cloning embryos for in vitro fertilization, somatic genetic therapy, or compensating young women for egg retrieval and transfer. The firestorm of controversy about reproductive cloning in the world has shown us how emotional the debate can be about a new form of human reproduction, such that the word "cloning" is almost too explosive to use in rational debate.

People today have been conditioned by media, religious leaders and ethicists to immediately associate increased parental choice about babies with eugenics, designer babies, slippery slopes, and even Nazi medicine. These associations, and their assorted charges, do not constitute good reasons but are thinly-disguised attempts to stop the back-and-forth dialectic of reasons.

Overall, and over the last century, North Americans and Europeans seem to fear choices about children of ordinary people, especially choices about the kinds of children those parents might want and create.

So what lesson does this brief history of assisted reproduction tell us about how any breakthrough toward an artificial human womb will be greeted? First, critics will decry the artificial womb as anti-family, the start of a slippery slope, an example of medical technology run amuck, and as a threat to traditional society. Second, the only real moral argument against the artificial womb is likely harm to the prospective baby.

4. The Artificial Womb and the Best Interests of the Child

Is ectogenesis in the best interests of the child? Wouldn't natural motherhood always be better? Once one starts to reflect on it, this is not necessarily so. Women with damaged or dysfunctional wombs will not be able to gestate children, and most of them either cannot or will not hire a surrogate. Besides surrogacy is not very efficient for most cases. So for some embryos, ectogenesis may be the only way they get gestated, and for some women, the only way an embryo from their egg will become a child.

Couldn't we use surrogates for such at-risk fetuses? Not often, because women willing to be surrogates are scarce, expensive, and not available on demand when a pregnant woman presents in crisis at the emergency room. Moreover, what about women with damaged wombs or no womb? We can always use new tools and should never bar any new tool from being created, especially when it enables us to start and preserve human life. Indeed, what could be more "pro-life"?

In discussing the best interests of the child here, we must tread carefully, because "good of the child" is a loaded, ambiguous phrase. The usual assumption made by conservative critics of assisted reproduction is that the ideal way to be born is to be a child of married, heterosexual parents who carefully plan the pregnancy. Any deviation from this idea, say, by introducing a third party as a sperm or egg donor, or surrogate, is held to harm the resulting child.

Thinking through what does not yet exist can be problematic for bioethics, which must be based on medical facts. Nevertheless, we can imagine that, if safe, the artificial womb might have several benefits for the fetus gestated in it.

First, some mothers during pregnancy use alcohol, cocaine, tobacco, and other substances likely to be harmful to the fetus. Because the mother's biological system is the same as the fetus', whatever risks the mother takes are also borne by the fetus. But the fetus is at a much more vulnerable stage than the mother, so the risks of harm from such substances may be greater. By raising the fetus in a uniform, stable, drug-free and controllable environment, the fetus is spared from risks associated with the mother using drugs.

For some babies, these risks can be considerable. Women who contract HIV may pass it to their fetuses, and even if AZT is used to block transmission of HIV from mother to fetus, AZT itself may harm the fetus. Of course, the artificial womb itself has risks. It could lose its source of electrical power, suffer a leak of fluids, or be mismanaged in any of a dozen ways. The question for consideration here will never be whether there is no risk of using an artificial womb but always whether the risks of such usage are outweighed by the benefits.

The above discussion focused on benefits to the fetus of removing toxins in its gestational environment but the flip side of that coin has the potential for even greater benefits. The same control that is possible that allows prevention of toxins entering the fetus's blood also allows for careful monitoring and study of the *best possible* nutrients for the fetus. That is, we might be able to change the gestational course for a poor baby of an alcoholic mother from being born addicted to alcohol and retarded to being born alcohol-free and with superior nutrition and oxygenation.

Yet another medical benefit of the artificial womb is that it would allow surgery to correct defects such as hydrocephaly (build-up of fluid inside the brain) or cleft palate. A surgeon could fix a defect in a spinal cord or heart valve much more easily than if she had to cut open a woman's uterus. Such in utero surgery is now done for some fetal defects, but it is dangerous and controversial. It would likely be much safer if it occurred inside an artificial womb.

5. The Artificial Womb and the Best Interests of the Mother

In the classic cases of fetal-maternal conflict, young physicians are often reminded that there are "two patients here, the mother and the child." Similarly, the artificial womb might have benefits for two patients, both the fetus and the mother. Sigmund Freud once famously remarked, "For women, biology is destiny." The artificial womb could change that.

One imaginative vision of how society might change from the artificial womb was given to us by Ursula K. Le Guin's novel of science fiction, *The Left Hand of Darkness*. In that book, not only women but also men have monthly cycles regulated by hormones, only in this world, gender is not fixed over time because humans alternate between cycles as men or women. However, if a human becomes pregnant during his female cycle, the human must stay female until the baby is gestated. From the mere fact that no human is biologically tied to gestation (a human can choose not to get pregnant, or stay pregnant, during a female cycle), many things change in this futuristic society. In particular, many sexist aspects of society change, since everyone is female half the time.

The artificial womb would free women from the tyranny of gestation. Although many women would undoubtedly choose to gestate their fetuses and they would celebrate their choice and believe it best for their fetus, others would not, so we can foresee some debate among women about the wisdom of using the new option. Nevertheless, it is hard to see why having a new option would not be in the best interests of women in general. Allowing more choice and freedom about when and how to gestate, and especially about *whether* to be a gestator at all, gives more flexibility to women, who often must balance conflicting demands of child-raising, careers, and pregnancy.

Perhaps one of the most compelling reason for using the artificial womb is where pregnancy conflicts with the health of the mother or where it might actually hurt or kill the mother. There are various medical conditions where nine months of pregnancy will likely render a women's health worse-off than before pregnancy.

Furthermore, artificial wombs remove age limits to gestation. In some ways, that might be its most radical implication. After her only existing child was unpredictably killed, a sixty year old woman might be able to have her previously-frozen embryo gestated in such a womb.

More controversially, a young female who was raped or the victim of incest, who did not want to gestate a fetus, could be allowed to have the fetus transferred to an artificial womb to be given up for adoption. This creates a fascinating prospect. Assume for the moment that artificial wombs are safe and assume that enough funds are available to create enough for any woman who wants to use them. Given those assumptions, then the widespread use of artificial wombs might significantly decrease the number of abortions because any woman pregnant against her wishes who did not want to abort could transfer her pregnancy to an artificial womb. Then the child could be adopted by any of the one-in-twelve childless couples in America today.

Of course this scenario makes a lot of controversial factual assumptions that may turn out to be false, for example, that the embryo/fetus would be easily transferable to an artificial womb. Nevertheless, the scenario does show that a new piece of medical technology might have unexpected implications. In this case, abortion would probably become harder to justify because now an alternative, pro-life choice would be an option to either death or the fetus or involuntary gestation.

6. Bonding

It is almost certain that, should extracorporeal gestation become practical, critics will claim that mother and child are harmed because of a lack of bonding. What exactly is bonding? It is the alleged biological connection developed between female gestator and fetus during nine months of pregnancy.

In the Baby M case in 1985 in New Jersey, feminists divided into pro- and anti-bonding camps. During gestation, birth, and during breast-feeding, gestator Mary Beth Whitehead claimed she had bonded with Baby M. She claimed that the contract she had signed was invalid, because she did not understand the metaphysical and psychological connection that would develop wither baby.

A lot of women philosophers and psychologists laid in passionately on both sides of this bonding dispute. New York City psychology professor Phyllis Chesler claimed that "children bond with their mothers in utero" and "suffer terribly in all kinds of ways when this bond is prematurely or abruptly terminated." One can only imagine the harm that Chesler would predict if no bonding at all occurred when a fetus was gestated in an artificial womb.

Philosopher Hillary Baber confronted Chesler, arguing that little evidence exists in the social sciences about bonding in primates. Interestingly, Baber argued this while pregnant herself, whereas Chesler has never borne a child. Baber also noted that some traditional mothers may have asserted a mystical bonding to the child in order to maximize the social evaluation of their contribution. Hence, we can predict that such women will see extracorporeal gestation as a threat to their own roles, lives, and values.

Some women can bear a baby, give it up, and feel nothing. Philosopher Christine Sistare claims that such women are neither "monsters" nor perverts. Nor, she says, are they deficient in any way, just normal. Indeed, the common phenomenon of postpartum depression argues against bonding. How could a woman feel like killing a baby she had metaphysically bonded to?

Many people generalized from the one case of Baby M to all of commercial surrogacy, and eighteen states outlaws this practice. But in California, commercial surrogacy has been going along quietly for nearly two decades. Anthropologist Helena Ragone enlightened us on this topic by actually interviewing women who had worked as surrogates, many of them from California. Surprisingly, most already were mothers and saw themselves in altruistic ways. The money allowed them to work in (what they saw as) their natural, God-given role: to create life, to be mothers, to help others. The other surprising result was that the surrogates didn't mind giving up the baby. The surrogates were sad at the ending of their role of pregnant mother and the feeling of being special to everyone because of it.

This sadness confirms a widely-reported result discovered by nurse-researcher Nancy Reame, who interviewed 10 (and only 10!) surrogates who had given birth a decade before. Six of the ten expressed some disappointment, not at having been surrogates but because the "relationship had been abandoned by the adoptive couple at the time of birth (for 3 women) or over time (for 3 women)." The disappointed six expected long-term contact with the adoptive couple, i.e. a continuation of their feeling of being extremely special to the couple as the surrogate, but this was very unrealistic.

Historical evidence also argues against the alleged strength of bonding. Aristocratic women used wet nurses after birth to breastfeed their newborns. If such aristocrats had bonded with their children, wouldn't they want to breastfeed themselves? If bonding were real, how could they so easily give away their babies for breastfeeding to a stranger?

A further point about bonding. Notice how much work is done in reproductive ethics by appeals to psychological harm. Whether we are discussing cloning or artificial wombs, critics frequently appeal to this quasi-empirical, secular claim to justify their opposition to a new option about reproduction.

Finally, we should not accept the equation bandied around of late that feminism equates with being anti-biotech. Just because *Our Body, Ourselves* co-editor Judy Norsigian can justify abortion but not research on embryos, does not mean she speaks for most feminists or most women.

7. Research with Extracorporeal Gestation

If are ever going to develop an artificial womb, research will have to be done. But how will such research ever occur? Obviously, if we can't use federal funds to experiment on human embryos, we won't be able to do so on human fetuses in such an environment. So then the research will have to be privately funded.

For thirty years, viability of lungs of the premature baby has been the absolute barrier to progress towards an artificial womb. Reports of success using liquids to substitute for the nutrients in the mother's placenta have usually been exaggerated. Until the infant can breathe outside the mother's womb, even with tiny respirators, it is not really viable outside that womb. Any real research in this area would have to attack this problem.

Here arises an interesting question: Could such research go forward in private companies right now? We also know that researchers in assisted reproduction clinics can now use human embryos to do research. No law regulates how private clinics can study human embryos, although no federal funds can be used for this purpose. This fact raises the question: could private researchers *right now* try to gestate human embryos in extracorporeal gestation? I do not see why they could not, but I know of no one trying to do so. Undoubtedly, this is a loophole that social conservatives will want to close down.

In any case, it will be very difficult to do the practical research necessary to prove extracorporeal gestation safe for human babies. Critics such as Thomas Murray of the Hastings Center echo fundamentalist theologian Paul Ramsey's claim that such research would be "unconsented-to" research on the unborn. While ectogenesis research subjects a fetus/baby to an experiment that lacks well-characterized risk without consent from the subject, what Ramsey and Murray fail to mention is that every advance now available in our Children's Hospitals has resulted from research that subjected babies to unconsented-to risk, often without well-characterized risk. It is the nature of brilliant innovation that not all risk can be understood in advance.

In the present political climate, it is inconceivable that government monies would fund such research. Under President George Bush's administration, we cannot even agree to fund research using human embryos, so you can imagine how controversial such research would be on third-trimester human fetuses.

Lung viability is the key to survival for premature babies, as it has been for over 32 years now according to the literature. If a fetus can breathe with the assistance of small respirators, it has a chance to live. But if it cannot breathe, even with assistance, it has little chance. It follows that the logical candidates for research would be on premature babies that lacked viable lung function, probably around 20 to 22 weeks of gestation.

Research on improving lung viability would focus on a liquid environment mimicking the nutrients, oxygenated blood, hormones, and antibodies of the mother's womb. Like ventricular-assist devices that are bridges to heart transplants, such an extracorporeal womb, would be a bridge to a NICU and tiny respirators.

Hence, the most likely start for research on extracorporeal gestation will be as therapeutic measures for dying, premature babies. This start may get researchers around the criticism that they are using fetuses as guinea pigs with the goal of sparing future women the chores of gestation.

It is likely that, long before an operative, efficient mechanical womb is available, animal models may be tried in last-ditch efforts. In some ways, a primate is a primate is a primate, and primate surrogates might be possible for some human fetuses, especially if the animal hosts were genetically modified to have immune systems compatible with surrogacy.

Such research would run up hard against a current taboo in our society and in medical research: that it would be horrible and wrong to implant a human fetus inside a non-human primate mother. But if this were in the best interests of the child, wouldn't it be right to do so?

8. Social Justice and the Artificial Womb

It is predictable that a safe, efficient artificial womb would be critiqued as creating a further divide between rich and poor, as now rich women would not need to bear children any more, only poor ones. Just as some rich models today, for fear of distorting their bodies, hire surrogates to bear embryos created from their eggs, e.g., Cheryl Tiegs, so rich women in the future would simply deposit their embryos in incubators and go back to their normal lives. But what about poor women, or women who lack medical coverage for this?

The generic answer is that we do not need to have a definitive answer to questions about distributive social justice to know that a thing is good or bad. Every innovation in electronic, medicine, pharmacology, aviation, or mechanics is potentially available more to people who can afford innovations that to people who cannot. The point of scientific progress is not to be a handmaiden to those who wish to create a perfectly egalitarian society.

More practically, because of the great benefit to the child, it is likely that medical insurance would indeed pay for artificial wombs. Although future savings from preventive medical interventions are often exaggerated, in the case of the artificial womb, this might be true. Especially if we consider benefits to fetuses/babies not exposed to alcohol, nicotine, or cocaine, and especially if we consider that such exposure is more common among low-income mothers than high-income mothers, then the artificial womb might not be a tool that created more social justice but the reverse.

9. Predictable Alarmist Critiques

If an artificial womb was successfully developed, or even if scientists began to study it, it is easy to imagine the hysterical cries that Jeremiahs would emit about such a new technology. It would be said to be an assault on the dignity of humanity, especially the "dignity of motherhood," a dehumanization of child-bearing, against God's will, an attack on the traditional family, and a psychological trauma for any baby born this way.

And of course, no bioethicist could talk about the artificial womb without mentioning the slippery slope. If gestation is made predictable and if humans are no longer needed for it, what is next? Ordering babies out of a catalogue? Ordering egg and sperm out of a J. Crew catalogue to be raised in an Orvis incubator delivered nine months later to rich parents on the other side of the planet? (It's fun to turn alarmist and see how easy it is to raise such specters!)

One can imagine the artificial womb being held up as a reductio ad absurdum of technology-out-of-control rather than as a benefit to women. Indeed, we can predict that critics would actually say that women will be harmed by the artificial womb by being deprived of the benefits of gestation, such as bonding and (ahem) "the deep metaphysical joy of fulfilling their biological function."

In conclusion, the possibility of ecotogenesis will alarm people and conservative critics will predict the worst outcomes from use of this practice, which they will never accept as safe. Nevertheless, under carefully chosen circumstances, ectogenesis might be in the best interests of a fetus and/or the woman who otherwise might have tried to gestate the fetus. Research may be most justified on dying, premature fetuses for whom no other options are available. Other objections to ectogenesis, involving bonding or just social allocation, seem too premature and speculative to be persuasive at this point.

NOTES

1. Stephanie Coontz, *The Way We Never Were: American Families and the Nostalgia Trap* (New York: Basic Books, 1992), p. 11–12.

Seven

ECTOGENESIS AND THE ETHICS OF CARE

Scott Gelfand

1. Introduction

It is not difficult to imagine a future in which ectogenetic technology will be available to gestate for the full term an embryo conceived through the use of in vitro fertilization. In other words, we might soon see the day when a woman's contribution to the birth of a live baby will be similar to that of a man, namely, each will only need to provide or donate gametes. Given that such technology might be only years away and has potentially far reaching moral and social implications, it is surprising that little research has been published on the moral permissibility of the use of ectogenetic technology or on how the use of this technology ought to be regulated, if at all.

In this chapter, I would like to take on this task. However, unlike most discussions of bioethics and biotechnology, I will not examine this issue from a rights perspective or a utilitarian perspective. Rather, I will utilize an ethics of care perspective. I have two primary goals in mind. First, I hope to provide some insights into a number of issues concerning the morality of ectogenesis, specifically, whether ectogenesis is ever morally permissible, whether ecto-genesis ought to be legally regulated, and how the advent of ectogenesis will affect the abortion debate. My second goal is to demonstrate that the ethics of care is useful in the realm of bioethics.

2. The Ethics of Care

Carol Gilligan, in her 1982 book, *In a Different Voice: Psychological Theory and Women's Development*, advances the thesis that in addition to the dominant *masculine* approaches to ethics, namely Kantian deontology and consequentialism, there is an alternative *feminine* approach: the ethics of care. Gilligan claims that her experimental studies reveal that when resolving moral dilemmas, men are more likely to utilize the aforementioned masculine approaches, which I (along with others) will refer to as the ethics of justice. She furthermore claims the ethics of care is more likely to be utilized by women to resolve these same dilemmas.[1] Subsequent to the publication of *In a Different Voice*, a number of theorists interested in ethical theory have advanced different formulations of the ethics of care and have questioned the role that the ethics of care can play in the moral life. Although most ethics of care proponents do believe that the ethics of care is useful in the private realm (issues related to family and friends), these same theorists, e.g., Marilyn Friedman and Virginia Held, claim that the ethics of justice is necessary for the public realm (issues related to business and government). [2] I beg to differ and suggest that an ethics of care may be a suitable approach for *both* the private and public realms. Significantly, Nel Noddings, who argued that the ethics of care is only applicable to the private realm in *Caring: A Feminine Approach Ethics and Moral Education*[3], is now coming to the view that the ethics of care can play a role in the public realm.[4]

In this chapter, I will explore whether the ethics of care might be employed to give us guidance when examining biomedical ethics issues that arise in *both* the private and public realms. Specifically, I will address whether the ethics of care might help us understand better if and when the use of ectogenesis is morally permissible in the private realm, whether the ethics of care might be useful to policy makers considering legislation regulating the use of ectogenesis and how the ethics of care might provide guidance to the issue of abortion, which takes on a new life when one considers the effect of ectogenesis on the abortion debate.

Before turning to the topic of ectogenesis, however, I would like to examine two different ethics of care formulations. The first, which Michael Slote calls the *morality of caring*, is a form of agent-based virtue ethics. I reject Slote's approach for a number of reasons, among them the fact that the morality of caring does not provide sufficient guidance when addressing moral questions. The second approach, which I support, is also a form of agent-based virtue ethics. However, as I will explain shortly, unlike Slote's approach, this second approach, which I call hypothetical-agent-based virtue ethics, does provide guidance.

3. Agent-Based Virtue Ethics, the Morality of Caring and Justice

In "The Justice of Caring" and *Morals From Motives*, Michael Slote attempts to demonstrate that the ethics of care is applicable to the public realm. Slote argues that the ethics of care is best conceived of as a virtue ethics theory or, specifically, what Slote calls an *agent-based* virtue ethics.[4] Agent-based virtue ethics, which is an approach inspired by the British Sentimentalists, specifically, Shaftesbury, Hutcheson, and Hume, dictates that an act's moral evaluation is determined *entirely* by the motives of the agent performing the act. Put simply, agent-based virtue ethics dictates that an act that expresses or flows from virtuous motives (or other character traits) is morally right, good, or admirable, and an act that expresses or flows from motives (or other character traits) far enough away from these virtuous motives (or character traits) is morally wrong, bad, or deplorable.

Agent-basing further dictates that moral evaluations of motives (or other character traits) are ethically basic or made at ground level. That is, judgments concerning whether a motive (or other character trait) is morally good or virtuous are made without regard to whether acting out of such a motive (or other character trait) brings about good consequences. Rather, a motive (or other character trait) is judged to be morally good just because it is fundamentally or inherently good.

An ethics of care conceived of as an agent-based virtue ethics begins with the assertion that care is, intuitively, a praiseworthy or morally good motive. For such an approach, the criterion of act assessment is (something like): an act is morally right if and only if it expresses, flows from, or reflects care (or a motive not too far from care). Slote calls this approach *the morality of caring*. According to the morality of caring, if an agent is performing an act that has the consequence of helping another, the act is morally right or good if and only if the agent is motivated by care (or a motive not too far from care). Accordingly, if the agent is motivated by a desire to somehow benefit (herself) and has no concern for the one being helped, the act is wrong. If, however, the agent's motive is care or concern for the one being helped, she performs a right act or acts rightly. Similarly, if an act has the consequence of hurting another, and the agent is motivated by care, the act is right.

In my "Hypothetical Agent-Based Virtue Ethics," I argue that Slote's approach is not without objection, but that it may, nevertheless, be a plausible approach to act evaluations.[6] But how can the morality of caring be applied to evaluations concerning the justice or lack thereof of laws, institutions, and societies? Slote suggests that we treat such evaluations in a way that is similar to or parallel to the way in which we treat the evaluation of acts. That is, in the same way that an agent-based approach grounded in care dictates that an act is right if and only if it expresses good motives (care or a motive not too far from care), agent-basing, when applied to the realm of justice, dictates that a law or institution is just if and only if it expresses good motives (care or a motive not too far from care). Slote calls this approach *the justice of caring*. But how can a law express good (or bad) motives? Slote answers this question by asserting that laws are really acts of legislators (or legislatures) and express motives in the same way that other acts express motives. In fact, some laws are called acts; e.g., the Stamp Act or the Tax Act of 1986. Accordingly, in order to determine whether a law is just, we must determine whether the legislators who voted for (or against) it were motivated by virtue (care or a motive not too far from care) when they voted. If they were motivated by care, then the resulting law is just, and if not, it is unjust. For example, consider a law mandating progressive taxation, that is, a tax structure that taxes those making a higher salary at a rate that is higher than the rate applied to those making a lower salary. According to Slote's justice of caring, if this law was passed by legislators whose votes were motivated by care, the law is just. If, however, the legislators were motivated by hatred of the wealthy (and were not concerned with how the law would affect those earning very little), the law is unjust.

As I explain in "The Ethics of Care and (Capital?) Punishment," one objection to Slote's morality of caring and other approaches to the ethics of care is that such approaches can be (and usually are) conceived of and formulated as partialistic moral theories.[7] That is, the morality of caring and other approaches to the ethics of care dictate that at the very least it is permissible, and it may be obligatory, for an agent to give precedence to the interests of her/his own family (and to a lesser extent her/his friends) over the interests of strangers. But if this is the case, then theoretical consistency dictates that lawmakers ought to care more for, or give precedence to the interests of, their families and friends when considering legislation. Yet, our common-sense intuitions dictate that laws passed by those whose behavior is motivated by a bias toward their own families at the expense of others are unjust.

Slote, who is aware of this objection, attempts to justify a caring lawmaker's shift to impartially when acting in the public or political realm. Slote points out that moral shifts are not foreign to common-sense morality. For example, common-sense morality dictates that an agent has a permission to favor her/his own projects as well as those who are near and dear to her/him, even when doing so is at a cost to overall optimality of results: "common-sense also tells us that when the stakes are high enough these just-mentioned permissions ... are displaced or superseded.... [I]f one's own personal and even one's family's flourishing would mean the extinction of one's entire ethnic group or country, one is no longer urged or permitted to pursue such flourishing." Essentially, Slote believes that a humanitarianism is aroused in an agent when large scale "humanitarian considerations enter the picture." Slote claims that a similar shift occurs when one goes from the private to the public realm. When one enters the public realm "the scale of action changes ... it is as if a person were somehow entrusted with the fate of a large number of individuals." In such cases, he concludes, "political roles should override considerations of personal or family advantage in those who have a deep and genuine love of their own country."[8]

A different way to defend the move from partiality in the private realm to impartiality in the public realm is to assert that intuitively, principles concerning what attitudes are appropriate or admirable when operating in the personal realm are different from those concerning what attitudes are appropriate or admirable when operating in the public realm. Such a move is particularly suited to agent-basing, given that the theorist must start by making claims about the intuitive moral goodness of character traits or motives and then assert that an act that expresses these character traits or motives is morally right or good. Perhaps one such claim is something like the following: Caring is a morally good or admirable motive, and in the personal realm partialistic caring is admirable (caring most about one's family and friends), and in the public realm impartialistic caring is admirable. Again, I believe that such a claim is, intuitively, plausible. An agent-based approach grounded in partialistic and impartialist caring might dictate that acts in the personal realm are morally right if and only if they express partialistic caring, and acts in the public realm are morally right if and only if they express impartialistic caring.

Although Slote's approach does reveal that it may be possible, in theory, to come up with a means of evaluating laws from an ethics of care perspective, his approach is open to a number of objections. First, as I point out in *The Ethics of Care and (Capital?) Punishment*, the justice of caring does not conceptually allow for the evaluation of the justice of laws before they are passed, that is, while they are being debated or examined.[9] This is the case because such evaluations are determined by the motives of the actual legislators voting for or against a statute. Because no one has yet voted, there are no motives to evaluate and we cannot, therefore, determine whether the law is just. If we were talking about acts, we might say that Slote's approach is not action guiding.

A second and related objection is that the justice of caring allows for identical pieces of legislation in relevantly similar societies to be evaluated differently. Let us again return to progressive taxation legislation. Suppose that the legislators in a given society who passed such legislation were motivated by care; they researched the economic literature and concluded that such legislation dramatically helps those at the lower end of the earning continuum and does little harm to those on the opposite end. According to the justice of caring, such a piece of legislation is just. Let us compare this with an identical piece of legislation that was passed by legislators motivated by hatred and selfishness. They voted for the statute because they hated those who earn a large salary and wanted to harm this group. They were totally unconcerned about their constituents and would not have supported the legislation if it did not somehow hurt large wage-earners. According to Slote's justice of caring, this piece of legislation is unjust. I contend that such an approach is, at the very least, counter-intuitive in that most of us believe that both statutes are either just or unjust. We might want to morally criticize the legislators whose votes were motivated by hatred and question whether they are worthy of being legislators, but this is a far cry from asserting that the legislation they passed is unjust.

Finally, justice of caring is open to an array of objections of a practical nature. To begin with, it is not only theoretically possible, but often times the case, that different legislators pass laws for different reasons. Consider a legislature, made up of one hundred legislators, that passes the above described taxation legislation by a vote of fifty-two to forty-eight. Let us further assume that the forty-eight who voted against the law did so solely out of concern for themselves. In addition, twelve of those who voted for the law despise those in poverty but despise even more those who are wealthy, and the fact that the law would hurt the high wage-earners was the primary or sole factor that motivated them to vote for the law. Like the behavior of those who voted against the law, the behavior of these twelve legislators does not express care or virtue. Finally, the remaining forty who voted for the law did so out of care or concern for the general public, both low and high wage earners. They did not want to hurt high wage earners, but concluded that the pain or loss they would suffer would be negligible, however, low wage-earners would gain significantly. In this scenario, the votes of only forty percent of the legislature were motivated by virtue. But forty out of fifty-two who voted for the bill, or seventy-seven percent of those who voted for, did so out of virtuous motives. Is this law just according to Slote? I'm not sure. A different possible breakdown of votes may be a difficulty for Slote's approach. Again, suppose that fifty-two legislators voted for the bill and forty-eight voted against it. What if the forty-eight who voted against the bill were motivated by virtue, twelve of the fifty-two who voted for it were also motivated by virtue, and the remaining forty who voted for the bill were not motivated by virtue? Is the law just? Again, I do not know what Slote would say about such a case.

4. Hypothetical-Agent-Based Virtue Ethics

Given the aforementioned objections to Slote's *justice of caring*, I suggest that we look at an alternative approach. I call this approach *hypothetical-agent-based virtue ethics*. Before discussing how hypothetical-agent-based virtue ethics can be applied to the realm of justice, I would like to briefly explain how it operates in the personal realm. As the name implies, hypothetical-agent-based virtue ethics is an approach that grounds evaluations of acts in the hypothetical acts of hypothetical agents. Specifically, hypothetical-agent-basing dictates that act is right if and only if it is the type of act that a hypothetical virtuous agent might perform. (By using the word "might" instead of "would" in this formulation, I implicitly assume that there is more than one possible act that a hypothetical agent might perform.) As is the case with standard or actualist agent-basing, when constructing a hypothetical-agent-based approach, the theorist must first determine what motives are praiseworthy and then assert that an act is right if and only if it is the type of act that might be performed by an agent acting out of these motives.

I want to point out that this formulation of hypothetical agent-basing is not an ideal observer theory. Ideal observer theories typically do not evaluate the observer's character, and they say nothing about the relationship between an agent's character and what is morally right. That is, ideal observer theories do not make the claim that the ideal observer has good character and because s/he has good character the act that s/he chooses is right. In fact, an ideal observer might realize that her/his own character is morally bad. So such views are not agent-based in any way.

Since I am interested in the ethics of care, I will assume that care is the best motive. Hence, according to hypothetical ABVE, an act is morally right if and only if it is the type of act that might be performed by one motivated by care. (By contrast, Slote's more familiar or standard ABVE treats acts as right if and only if they reflect actual good motives on the part of the actual agent.) If we assume that a law is an act of a legislature, then we can say that a law is just if and only if it is the type of law that might be passed by hypothetical caring legislators.

Notice that hypothetical-agent-based virtue ethics is not open to the objections I leveled against Slote's justice of caring. Since a law is just if and only if a hypothetical caring legislator might vote for it, we are not left with the counter-intuitive result of the possibility of two identical laws in relevantly similar societies being evaluated differently. If a statute is of the type that caring legislators might support, it is just, regardless of the actual motives of the legislators voting for or against the law. In addition, since the motives of the actual legislators are not relevant to the justice of a law, this approach is not open to the objection leveled against Slote's justice of caring concerning the different possible break down of votes for or against a piece of legislation.

Finally, hypothetical-agent-basing does give us guidance as to whether or not a law is just; that is, unlike Slote's approach, hypothetical agent-basing does not require that a law be voted on before it can be evaluated. We can determine whether a law is just by ascertaining whether caring legislators *might* vote for it. But this last is premised on the claim that we can, in fact, ascertain or determine what types of statues caring legislators might support. I believe we can do so and will now explain why I believe this is the case.

Historically, virtue ethicists have suggested that we look at role models or moral paradigms in order to determine what types of acts (or character traits) are morally good. Rosalind Hursthouse, for example, says that we might formulate virtue ethics as follows: "An action is right if and only if it is what a virtuous agent would characteristically (i.e. acting in character) do in the circumstances."[10] Harold Alderman makes a similar claim and argues that the best starting point for an ethical theory is the character of a moral exemplar or outstanding moral individual. Alderman claims that some of the Socratic dialogues were written by Plato in order to demonstrate to the reader how a virtuous agent might act. He further claims that Aristotle believed that we could act morally if we acted like Aristotle, who conceived of himself as a moral exemplar.[11]

Care ethicists have asserted that the paradigmatic relationship is that between a mother and child. But I see no reason why we should not extend this to both parents, thus I suggest that we use caring parents in a nuclear family as the paradigm and attempt to determine how they might act in a given situation. Specifically, I propose that we use caring parents in a nuclear family as a heuristic devise in order to determine how a caring legislator might respond to questions concerning potential legal regulations. Elsewhere I've written about criminal punishment and suggested that in order to determine whether legislation concerning punishment is just or appropriate, we should attempt to determine how caring parents would respond to violations of rules within a family.[12] Presumably, when considering punishment, caring parents would be concerned with, among other things, protecting their children from harms resulting from future possible violations of rules, teaching their children that violating rules is wrong and restoring the relationships that might be injured as a result of rule violations. Thus, by using the family as a model we learn that caring legislators ought to have similar concerns and would support legislation that addresses these concerns. As I will explain later, a similar approach can be used to determine whether legislation regulating the use of ectogenesis is appropriate or just.

5. Hypothetical-Agent-Based Virtue Ethics and Ectogenesis

So what does a hypothetical-agent-based virtue ethics grounded in care tell us about the moral permissibility of ectogenesis? First I will attempt to determine what hypothetical-agent-basing tells us about the moral permissibility of utilizing ectogenesis in cases related to the private realm, that is, cases in which a women (and/or a man) are presented with the opportunity to gestate a fetus in an artificial womb. I will then examine cases related to the public realm, specifically cases concerned with legislation regulating (or prohibiting) the use of ectogenesis. In section 6, I discuss how an ethics of care might affect discussions concerning abortion and the relationship between abortion and ectogenesis.

A. Ectogenesis in the Private Realm

Recall the criterion of act evaluation for a hypothetical-agent-based approach grounded in care: an act is right if and only if it is the type of act that a caring agent might perform. Accordingly, in order to determine whether utilizing ectogenesis is ever permissible (or even obligatory) we must attempt to determine if a caring agent might utilize ectogenesis. I think the least controversial case would be one in which an agent desires to have a genetically related child, but is unable to gestate a fetus.

For example, consider an agent who has fertile eggs but no longer has a uterus. The only ways in which she will be able to have a genetically related child is by undergoing *in vitro fertilization* and utilizing either a surrogate or ectogenetic technology. If ectogenesis has no (or very limited) negative effects on the health and well-being of the fetus (and the agent is unable to secure the services of a surrogate), it seems clear that a caring agent might choose to use it and that ectogenesis is, in such a case, morally permissible. After all, the agent is motivated by a desire to have a (genetically related) child, and such a desire is not (typically) a manifestation or expression of a lack of care.

If there is, however, a surplus of adoptable children and the agent insists on utilizing ectogenesis to have her own genetically related child, then the act may reflect a lack of caring. But such an act is not wrong because the agent wants to use ectogenesis. Rather, it is wrong because the agent's behavior expresses a lack of concern for the well-being of the potential adoptees. If she insisted on a surrogate to carry her child it would be equally wrong. Accordingly, I conclude that in cases in which one uses ectogenesis even when there is a surplus of available children, it is not the use of ectogenesis that is wrong. In cases in which such a surplus does not exist, ectogenesis does not reflect a lack of care and is, I believe, morally permissible.

Of course there may be health or developmental problems associated with ectogenesis. For example, fetuses gestated in an artificial womb may not receive the same sorts of stimulation or nutrition that they would receive from a natural womb. If this is the case, then presumably a caring agent would be more inclined to seek out a surrogate as opposed to opting for ectogenesis, and ectogenesis would be wrong.

In addition, it is conceivable that those who use an artificial womb do not bond with the future child in the same way that those who naturally gestate a future child bond with it. This may be true, but many adoptive parents seem to develop quite strong bonds with the children they adopt, even though they do not gestate these children. Also, Shulamith Firestone, in *The Dialectics of Sex*, asserts that a woman "who undergoes a nine-month pregnancy is likely to feel that the product of all that pain and discomfort 'belongs' to her."[13] This, Firestone suggests, leads to an unhealthy possessiveness and negatively affects the mother child relationship. So, although the effect of ectogenesis on mother-child bonding may be a concern for a caring agent, at this point I do not think we have enough information to conclude that a caring agent would reject ectogenesis because of its effect on this bond. Notice that these matters are empirically grounded, and until we have more evidence it will be impossible to determine the permissibility of ectogenesis, but it does appear that under certain circumstances ectogenesis is permissible.

What about those cases in which an agent wants to utilize ectogenesis in order to avoid all or some of the side effects of pregnancy, such as morning sickness, frequent urination, weight gain, etc...? It appears that such an agent is acting out of self-concern. This may be true, but it does not necessary follow that one acting out of self-concern is also expressing a lack of care for others. Clearly, an agent who deeply cares for her fetus and future child may at the same time want to avoid the aforementioned effects of pregnancy. Thus, it appears that ectogenesis may be permissible in these sorts of cases.

Of course, if ectogenesis exposes the fetus to more potential harm than natural gestation, but the agent wants to use it nevertheless in order to avoid a minor inconvenience like stretchmarks, we might correctly conclude that she is expressing a deficiency of care and such an act would be wrong. Again, we need to obtain additional empirical data concerned with how ectogenesis affects future children in order to determine whether using ectogenesis in these types of cases is permissible.

Might an agent be morally required to use ectogenesis? This again will depend on, among other things, how ectogenesis will affect the fetus and the life of the future child. If, for example, we discover that ectogenesis is *much* healthier for the fetus than natural gestation, then presumably a caring agent would opt for using ectogenetic technology. This is the case, even if the future mother has a strong desire to experience pregnancy and delivery.

Although I have not provided easy, clear-cut answers as to whether ectogenesis is permissible in the private realm, I want to stress that the preceding discussion demonstrates that the ethics of care is capable of giving us guidance with this issue. Furthermore, it is not clear that act-utilitarianism or (what I believe are plausible forms of) deontology provide any more guidance than does the ethics of care. A utilitarian will tell us that ectogenesis is right if and only if it maximizes the good. But if we ask her/him to tell us whether it will, in fact, maximize the good, s/he will likely tell us s/he does not know. Of course, as Eugene Bayles points out, this is not necessarily an objection to utilitarianism.[14] Similarly, if we look to Ross's deontology for guidance with the ectogenesis issue, we will discover we have a number of competing prima facie duties, including competing duties of beneficence and justice. Finally, it is not clear to me that Kantian deontology fares any better with the issue of ectogenesis than does act-utilitarianism or Ross's deontology, but that is a difficult issue that I will leave for another time.

B. Ectogenesis in the Public Realm

I will now move to the public realm and attempt to determine what types of legislation or regulations might be justified by a hypothetical-agent-based approach grounded in care. As stated in section 4, hypothetical-agent-based virtue ethics dictates that a law is just if and only if it is the type of law that caring legislators might support. What types of legislation aiming at regulating ectogenesis might be supported by caring legislators? Would caring legislators permit the use of ectogenesis in any circumstances?

As discussed above, ectogenetic technology might permit those who are physically incapable of carrying a fetus to term to obtain a genetically related child. On its face, this seems to be a good thing, and I believe that if this were the only instance in which ectogenesis would be used, caring legislators would support making this opportunity available. But there are other possible ways in which ectogenesis might be used.

The availability of ectogenesis may seriously affect attitudes and policies concerning employee/employer rights. Hard battles have been fought with the goal of ensuring that women will not be penalized or terminated for missing work due to pregnancy. With ectogenetic technology available, employers might *strongly encourage* women to utilize ectogenesis and threaten penalties for a woman's failure to do so. It is not difficult to conceive of an employer, a managing partner of law firm, for example, who would see no difference between a woman missing work because she chooses to naturally gestate and carry her fetus to term and a woman who misses work because she chooses to spend her afternoons in a museum. The managing partner might plausibly claim (and even believe) that each of these women is making the choice to sacrifice her office productivity in order to pursue other interests.

Should there be regulations or legislation prohibiting employers from penalizing employees who choose to naturally gestate a future child? Employers who coerce their employees to use ectogenesis limit their employees' range of choice. Clearly, many women believe that their well-being would be decreased if they were to lose the opportunity to choose freely whether to naturally gestate their future offspring. A managing partner may agree that coercing women to utilize ectogenesis is harmful to women, yet at the same time also assert that not coercing them to do so hurts the law firm. Thus, it appears that one considering whether to regulate ectogenesis must decide whether the interests of the employers or those of pregnant women ought to take priority.

Given these competing interests, would a caring legislator support legislation permitting or restricting ectogenesis? As I mention earlier in this chapter, elsewhere I suggest that we use caring parents in a nuclear family as a heuristic device to help us determine how caring legislators might respond to questions of public morality and justice. Thus, we need to find an analogous situation in a family setting and attempt to determine how caring parents might act in this situation.

In order to describe an analogous case, it will be helpful to keep in mind what the caring legislator might be thinking. Presumably, this legislator is attempting to determine whether the power of employers to coerce the use of ectogenesis should be limited. Such a limitation would preserve the well-being of women but hurt employers' profitability. No limitations, in the alternative, would preserve the employers' profitability but allow employers to coerce women to use ectogenesis and thereby harm women, who as a class, I will assume, have been disadvantaged in various ways in our society. On the face of it, a caring legislator would be torn.

So let us turn to the family and attempt to construct an analogous case. Consider a parent who owns a family business that employs two of her/his children, including Sally, who is the eldest daughter, and Katie, who is the youngest daughter, and who plans to naturally gestate and deliver her own future child. Since Sally is the eldest and has worked for the company longer than Katie, she is above Katie on the managerial hierarchy; in fact, she is the senior manager of the company, excepting her parent, who leaves most operational decisions to Sally. Katie is second to Sally. Imagine that the parent discovers that Sally has told Katie that if she, Katie, does not use a surrogate to gestate her future child, she (Katie) will be terminated. For the sake of discussion, let us assume that the business will suffer some financial loss but is doing well and will not be bankrupted if Katie takes the normal leave-time associated with gestation and delivery. Let us further assume that Katie has wanted to get pregnant and gestate her future child for a number of years; however, only recently has technology become available such that she can conceive. In addition, let us assume that Sally was hoping to go to graduate school in the near future and realize a long-held dream but will not be able to do so if Katie takes the leave-time associated with natural gestation and delivery. Finally, let us assume that Sally has had a storybook life, whereas Katie has had to contend with many difficulties. Sally was popular while growing up and was a good student. She knew from a young age that she wanted to go into the family business, and when she did so excelled. Katie, on the other hand, was unpopular and never did well in school. In addition, she decided to go to work for the family business because she could not find alternative employment.

So how would the parent react when s/he discovers that Sally threatened to terminate Katie if Katie does not use a surrogate? I suggest that most of us would expect a caring parent to intervene and reverse Sally's order. In fact, I suggest that a caring parent would be outraged. This is the case, I think, because the caring parent would recognize that gestating one's own fetus for the full term is quite important to Katie. Although the parent would likely identify with Sally's desire to increase (or limit any decrease in) the business's profitability and her desire to attend graduate school, a caring parent would recognize that Katie has had a difficult life and would desire to provide her the opportunity to achieve one of her dreams. After all, Sally has realized many of her own dreams and goals. Finally, if Sally tried to convince her parents that it would maximize overall well-being to require Katie to use the surrogate, the parent would be appalled, as would most of us. The parent would likely assert that unlike Sally, Katie has had to contend with many difficulties in her life, and that if we can make her life better in this instance, we ought to do so. The parents would not even begin to calculate which option would maximize the good, and those of us who approve of the parent's position do so because we believe that a caring parent ought not attempt to maximize well-being in these sorts of cases. It is important to keep in mind that the parent is acting impartially with respect to her/his concern for her/his daughters. That is, s/he does not believe that Katie's well-being ought to take precedence over Sally's well-being; rather, s/he believes that Katie has had fewer opportunities and successes in her life and when an opportunity presents itself it should be preserved.

With this example in mind, we turn to the legislator considering whether to regulate ectogenesis. Like the parent, the legislator must decide whether to limit a business's freedom to pursue profit and other goals in order to preserve an employee's freedom to choose, without penalty, between gestating her own child or using some alternative means. If a caring parent would conclude that one's interest in gestating one's own future child ought to take precedence (within reason) over the financial and other interests of a business and would attempt to secure her/his child's opportunity to gestate her/his future child, then presumably a caring legislator ought to act similarly and support legislation restricting an employer's right to limit her/his employees' freedom to naturally gestate a future child.

Accordingly, such legislation, according to the ethics of care approach I am proposing, would be just and good. Of course, in the case above, I make it clear that Katie has had less opportunity than Sally. Thus, my claim that such legislation is just depends on the claim that women have less opportunity (and therefore success) than men have in contemporary society. If this assumption is incorrect, then perhaps such legislation is not justified. Nevertheless, I hope it is becoming clear that an ethics of care is capable of helping us address bioethics issues related to both the private and public realms.

A second issue related to the availability of ectogenesis is insurance related. It is not inconceivable that the use of ectogenesis will become so widespread that it will be less expensive than natural gestation and delivery. After all, delivery of the baby will be much less invasive and time consuming than natural delivery. There will be no need for caesarian sections or chance of premature delivery. In addition, there will be no need for hospital stays for expectant mothers and those who have given birth. Might insurance companies employ financial pressures to exert people to use ectogenesis, such as not covering pregnancies or deliveries when a woman does not use ectogenesis? Should there be legislation restricting insurance companies from exerting these financial pressures?

Again, I suggest that we look to the family in order to determine how caring legislators might respond to these concerns. For the sake of this example, I will stipulate that ectogenesis is no safer for the future child than natural gestation and delivery. I will complicate matters by dropping this stipulation shortly.

Consider two forty year-old twins, Becky and Cindy, each of whom does not have health insurance. However, the siblings share a large trust fund, which is expected to pay for, among other things, the twins' health care expenses. Let us further assume that the siblings are co-trustees of the fund and that any withdrawals from the fund must be approved by both sisters. Finally, let us imagine that Becky (who has been disadvantaged throughout her life like Katie in the previous example) wants to get pregnant and naturally gestate and deliver her own future child. Cindy, when she hears of Becky's plans, investigates and discovers that the pregnancy and/or delivery may be costly due to potential complications associated with Becky's age. Cindy therefore concludes that it is unlikely that the cost will be more than ten thousand dollars, but that the risk of a high cost pregnancy and delivery, which could be twenty or thirty times as expensive as a normal pregnancy and delivery, can be almost eliminated if Becky uses a younger surrogate to carry her future child. How might Cindy's and Becky's parents react if they discover that Cindy will not sign off on the funds that Becky needs to naturally gestate and deliver her future child.

Assuming that natural gestation and delivery will not expose the sisters to *extreme* financial risk, I suggest that the parents will be outraged and will attempt to block Cindy's refusal to sign-off on the withdrawal of funds. Like the previous case, the parents will not calculate utility. Rather, they will recognize that preserving Becky's freedom to make reproductive choices is more important than saving money, even if preserving the opportunity to make such choices will expose their daughters to some financial risk. After all, they recognize that Cindy has had a good life with many opportunities, whereas Becky has had to contend with many difficulties and obstacles.

With this scenario in mind, we can transition to the question of how caring legislators might respond if insurance companies financially coerce women to use ectogenesis. Presumably, they will recognize how important it is for some women, who as a class have been disadvantaged in society, to have the opportunity to choose whether to naturally gestate and deliver their own future children and will, therefore, restrict insurance companies freedom to coerce women in the ways suggested earlier. Of course, if permitting women to naturally gestate and deliver their future children would bankrupt the insurance companies, we may have a different result.

Let us complicate matters by dropping the stipulation made in the previous example. Let us assume that ectogenesis would not only be less costly than natural gestation and delivery, but that it would be safer for both the future child and the woman who would otherwise carry the future child. This may not be a stretch given that ectogenesis would in all likelihood protect the fetus from second-hand smoke, alcohol, and an unhealthy diet. In fact, it may be the case that ectogenesis could provide a diet that is healthier for the future child than any diet adhered to by a pregnant woman. In addition, ectogenesis may be safer for the mother than natural delivery for obvious reasons. Finally, as Firestone pointed out, ectogenesis may lead to a healthier mother-child bond. Of course, many would deny Firestone's claim, but let us assume it is true for the sake of discussion.

With these factors in mind, let us return to Becky and Cindy. If Cindy was coercing Becky to use a surrogate because it was considerably safer and psychologically healthier for the future child, then it is not so clear that her parents would be outraged if they discovered that Cindy was not willing to release the funds that Betsy would need to naturally gestate and deliver her future child. In fact, it may be the case that they would support such a decision.

I conclude that whether a legislator should permit insurance companies to financially coerce women to use ectogenesis would depend, to some extent, on how ectogenesis would affect the health and well-being of the future child. Clearly, when more empirical evidence concerning these issues becomes available, legislators will need to study it in order to know whether to restrict insurance companies' right to coerce its use.

6. Abortion and Ectogenesis

Although a thorough discussion of abortion is beyond the scope of this chapter, I would like to explain briefly both how ectogenesis may dramatically affect the abortion debate and how the ethics of care may shed some insights into the issue of abortion in an ectogenetic world.

Those who believe abortion is morally permissible rely on a number of different arguments. I would like to look at two of the most popular. What both these arguments have in common is that they conceive of the abortion debate as a conflict between the right to life of the fetus and the right to bodily autonomy of a (pregnant) woman. Those who believe abortion is morally permissible, regardless of which of these two arguments they endorse, resolve this conflict in favor of the woman's right to bodily autonomy. Opponents of abortion resolve this conflict in favor of the fetus. As I will explain shortly, ectogenesis may alter the outcome of both of these arguments.

The first type of argument in support of the moral permissibility of abortion, which Leslie Cannold refers to as a "severance" theory,[15] is advocated by, among others, Judith J. Thomson in her essay, "A Defense of Abortion."[16] Advocates of this type of argument support the claim that abortion is permissible by arguing that a woman's right to autonomy extends to the right to remove a fetus from her own body or disconnect herself from a fetus, even if the fetus is a person and doing so will kill this person. Thomson claims that this type of argument allows us to circumvent the issue of whether a fetus is human. But for the sake of argument, she assumes it is human.

In her well-known violinist example, Thomson asks the reader to imagine that s/he wakes up one day and discovers that s/he is in a hospital bed with tubes going to and from her/his body and that of a famous violinist. The reader is told that the violinist will die if the reader chooses to unhook her/himself from the violinist. Thomson assumes that most readers will agree with her intuition that it would be morally permissible for the reader to disconnect her/himself from the violinist, even though the violinist will die. Thomson argues that abortion is permissible in the same way that it is permissible to unhook the violinist, even though doing so entails the foreseeable, but unintended, consequence of the death of the fetus. However, Thomson clearly states that if the violinist somehow lives, it would be impermissible to reach around and "slit his throat."[17] Similarly, she asserts that if the fetus somehow survives after you disconnect yourself from it, you have no right to "secure the death of the unborn child."[18]

The second type of argument in support of the permissibility of abortion, which I call developmental theories, are advanced by, among others, Mary Ann Warren. Warren proposes five criteria for personhood and concludes that a fetus (at least a young, undeveloped fetus) does not meet these criteria and is not, therefore, a person.[19] Since a person's right to bodily autonomy usually trumps a non-person's right to life, an agent, who is a person, has a right to abort and thereby kill a fetus or non-person.

The development of partial ectogenetic technology may have an effect on both severance and developmental arguments. If, as Thomson and others point out, a woman has a right to disconnect herself from a fetus but does not have a right to secure the death of the fetus, and if ectogenetic technology (and related technology to remove non-invasively the fetus from the womb) will allow for the preservation of the life of the fetus, then abortion (which has the consequence of killing the fetus) may not be justifiable. Of course, it does not follow that it will be wrong to undergo a termination of pregnancy (which does not lead to the death of the fetus) and place the fetus in an artificial womb. Recall that Thomson assumes, for the sake of argument, that the fetus is a human being. If a fetus is not human, then it may be permissible, depending on the moral status of a fetus, to abort a fetus even if ectogenetic technology (and related technology to remove non-invasively the fetus from the womb) is available. Thus, as I point out elsewhere, the advent of ectogenetic technology (and related technology to remove non-invasively the fetus from the womb) will require those who propose severance theories to determine the moral status of a fetus, an undertaking they hoped to avoid.[20] Is it more like a tumor, an ant, or a two-day old baby? Depending on how one answers this question, abortion may or may not be permissible.

I am not sure how the availability of partial ectogenesis will affect developmental arguments in support of abortion. Even if the fetus is not a human being, it does not necessarily follow that it is permissible to kill it for any reason. Most of us would agree that it is wrong to kill a chimpanzee, if the reason for doing so is petty, say the desire to discover how a chimpanzee tastes. On the other hand, many would agree that it is permissible to kill a fish or a deer in order to see how it tastes. Thus, in order to determine whether abortion will be permissible when ectogenetic technology (and related technology to remove non-invasively the fetus from the womb) becomes a reality, those who rely on developmental arguments will have to determine the moral status of a human fetus. Is it more like a chimpanzee or more like a fish or deer? As stated above, those who advance severance theories will have to make the same determination.

I contend that the ethics of care might be in a good position to address this issue. Much of what follows is borrowed from Michael Slote's unpublished manuscript entitled *Moral Sentimentalism*.[21] Although the following discussion is brief and does not even begin to do justice to Slote's proposed theory, I believe it is adequate for the purpose of this section.

In *Moral Sentimentalism*, Slote proposes an ethics of care that is grounded in *empathic* caring. Slote, citing the work of Martin Hoffman, claims that those who have a normally developed sense of empathy are pre-disposed to empathize and identify with the other. Although empathic identification does not deprive the agent of her/his own identity, it does allow the agent to feel what the other is feeling. Slote argues that an ethics of empathic caring offers both an explanation and a justification for many of our common-sense moral intuitions. For example, many care ethicists believe that our obligations to family and friends are stronger than our obligations to strangers halfway around the world. Perhaps this is the case, Slote suggests, because an agent with a normally (or fully) developed sense of empathy will naturally feel more empathy toward family and friends than s/he will toward strangers. If, as Slote claims, empathic care is a fundamentally good motive and an act is right if and only if it flows from or expresses empathic care, then we can explain why caring more for family and friends is justified and good (or right). After all, we can and do empathize (and identify) with family and friends more than we do with strangers.

Slote suggests that we can get new insights into the abortion debate, especially the question concerning the moral status of the fetus, by employing his ethics of empathic caring. In order to determine the moral status of a fetus, we must attempt to determine how an agent with a fully developed sense of empathy would respond to (and identify with) a fetus.

If, as Slote tentatively points out, many of us can and do empathize and identify with a newborn more deeply than we empathize with an embryo, then our obligations to fetuses are not as great as those to newborns. But even if this is the case, it does not necessarily follow that we have no obligations to fetuses. In order to determine what these obligations are, we must determine how one with a fully developed sense of empathy would respond to the potential death of a fetus. It may be the case that one with a normally developed sense of empathy cannot empathically identify with an early embryo, which is, after all, a clump of undifferentiated cells. If this is the case, then we have few or no obligations to an early embryo and abortion may be permissible even if ectogenesis is available. As the fetus develops and begins to resemble us, however, we will likely have the capacity to empathically identify with it more, and our obligations become more strict. This may entail an obligation to use ectogenesis when terminating a pregnancy.

But I am not at all sure that this analysis of our capacity to empathize with an undeveloped fetus is correct. Perhaps John Noonan, whose essay, "Responding to Persons: Methods of Moral Argument in Debate over Abortion," which discusses the relationship between empathy and fetal rights, is correct.[22] Noonan argues that an agent can and should empathize with the fetus and recognize that the fetus is part of "the family of man." If Noonan is correct, then presumably abortion will be wrong when ectogenesis become available. Given this disagreement, if we want to determine whether abortion will be permissible in a world with the availability of ectogenesis, we will have to do more research into how an agent with a fully developed sense of empathy will respond to the possibility of the death of a fetus.

7. Conclusion

Throughout much of this chapter I have not attempted to provide clear-cut answers to the moral questions associated with the advent of ectogenesis. I do claim that ectogenesis may be permissible in some cases and that we should be ready to enact legislation to preserve a woman's freedom to choose to naturally gestate her future offspring, but even these claims are premised on empirical assumptions that are currently unsupported because the evidentiary data is unavailable. I do hope, however, that I have demonstrated that the ethics of care is in a better position than many realize to help us better understand, gather insights, and make progress with moral questions related to ectogenesis in particular and bioethics more generally speaking in both the public and private realms. Perhaps this is all we can ask from a moral theory.

NOTES

1. Carol Gilligan, *In A Different Voice* (Cambridge, Mass.: Harvard University Press, 1982), especially chap. 2.

2. Marilyn Friedman, *What are Friends For?* (Ithaca, N.Y.: Cornell University Press, 1993), pp. 87–88; Virginia Held, *Feminist Morality* (Chicago: University of Chicago Press, 1993), p. 76.

3. Nel Noddings, *Caring: A Feminine Approach Ethics and Moral Education* (Berkeley, Cal.: University of California Press, 1984).

4. Nel Noddings, *Starting at Home: Caring and Social Policy* (Berkeley Cal.: University of California Press, 2002).

5. Michael Slote, "The Justice of Caring," *Social Philosophy and Policy* 15 (1998), pp. 171–195; *Morals From Motives* (Oxford: Oxford University Press, 2003).

6. Scott Gelfand, "Hypothetical Agent-Based Virtue Ethics," *Southwest Philosophy Review* 11 (2000), pp. 85–94.

7. Scott Gelfand, "The Ethics of Care and (Capital?) Punishment," *Law and Philosophy* 23 (2004), pp. 593–614.

8. *The Justice of Caring*, pp. 184–186.

9. "The Ethics of Care of (Capital?) Punishment."

10. Rosalind Hursthouse, "Normative Virtue Ethics," in *How Should One Live? Essays on the Virtues*, ed. Roger Crisp (New York: Oxford University Press, 1996), p. 22.

11. Harold Alderman, in "By Virtue of a Virtue," *Review of Metaphysics* 36 (1982), pp. 127–153.

12. "The Ethics of Care and (Capital?) Punishment."

13. Shulamith Firestone, *The Dialectic of Sex* (New York: William Morrow and Company, 1970), p. 232.

14. Eugene Bayles, "Utilitarianism: Account Of Right-Making Characteristics Or Decision-Making Procedure?" *American Philosophical Quarterly* 8 (1971), pp. 257–265.

15. Leslie Cannold, "Women, Ectogenesis, and Ethical Theory," *Journal of Applied Philosophy* 12 (1995), p. 55 [this volume, p. 47].

16. Judith Jarvis Thomson, "A Defense of Abortion," *Philosophy and Public Affairs* 1 (1971), pp. 47–66.

17. Thomson, p. 66.

18. Thomson, p. 66.

19. Mary Anne Warren, "On the Moral and Legal Status of Abortion," *Monist* 57 (1973), pp. 43–61.

20. Scott Gelfand, "Marquis: A Defense of Abortion?" *Bioethics* 15 (2001), pp. 135–145.

21. Michael Slote, *Moral Sentimentalism*, unpublished manuscript.

22. John Noonan, "Responding to Persons: Methods of Moral Argument in Debate over Abortion," *Theology Digest* 21 (Winter 1973), pp. 91–107.

Eight

OF MACHINE BORN? A FEMINIST ASSESSMENT OF ECTOGENESIS AND ARTIFICIAL WOMBS

Maureen Sander-Staudt

Ectogenesis poses the end to the fact that up to this point in history, all human life has been "of woman born." Scientists predict that within the next 30 years, artificial wombs will become a reality. If this technology is perfected the day could come when conception, gestation and birth is a controlled process regulated by machines in labs or hospitals, and womb transplants are as common caesarian sections. Among other things this social development promises to significantly alter women's physical and social connections to pregnancy and birth.

In this chapter ectogenesis is examined from the perspective of feminist ideals about justice and the good in order to highlight some of the promise and problems of this technology. First, I explain why artificial womb technology should not be ethically assessed without sensitivity to sex and gender. Second, I use the disparate frameworks of liberal, radical, and cultural feminism to argue that artificial wombs have the potential to both improve and harm the social status of women in the United States. Finally, although there can be no singular feminist position with regards to ectogenesis, I argue that radical, cultural, and eco feminism make an ethically important departure from liberal feminist analyses by emphasizing the intersubjectivity of a mother and fetus during pregnancy—an emphasis that I assert is central to the full ethical assessment of artificial womb technologies. Specifically, an ethics of care that draws from these feminist perspectives is used to analyze and critique ectogenesis by showing how it is problematic on both scientific and cultural grounds. Despite the ways that ectogenesis might offer "therapeutic" options to many individuals including women and children, a feminist ethics of care reveals some potential dangers associated with the development of the artificial womb.

1. Ectogenesis is a Gender Issue

Ectogenesis is a word that many dictionaries omit, reflecting that this concept is yet to be fully defined. But the root words are readily definable: "ecto" means outer or outside, and "genesis" means origin or start. But what is missing from this simple definition is exactly who or what is starting outside of whom or what. This definition excludes all human reference, and thus obscures the ethical perimeters of this debate. The term "artificial womb" does not do much better since it also conceals the human persons likely to be directly affected by the technology in question. The obfuscation of human persons by the language of ectogenesis may reflect the general ability of ectogenic technology to reconfigure fetal gestation such that the traditional human relationship is altered or reduced. For the sake of my argument, then, let me offer my own definition: ectogenesis is a technological process whereby an embryo or fetus is biologically nurtured outside of a mother's body for the length of the entire gestational process, from conception to birth. This is to be distinguished from the act of incubating a child who is born prematurely, which I will refer to as partial ectogenesis, or more generally, artificial womb technology (AWT). The virtue of these definitions is not just that they highlight the general human elements of ectogenesis, but also the special connection that women and children bear to these technologies. However, as later will become apparent, ectogenesis still needs clarification as artificial womb technology promises to alter the precise moment and meaning of "birth."

The achievement of ectogenesis is likely to evolve from bridging the gap between in vitro fertilization and the incubation of premature infants, a gap currently of around 20 weeks. One of the most recent developments is "Freddy the Frog," what is being called part of an "artificial womb" for the improved treatment of premature infants. In addition to the control of light, temperature, air, and nutrients, babies are tucked in a snuggle-up pack and a curved rod is placed around them, mimicking the abdominal wall of their mothers.[1] By providing boundaries this "womb" allows the infants to save their energy, resulting in calmer vital signs and improved growth. Studies show that this treatment results in fewer days in the hospital and on respirators for children. Along with the pack, many doctors also recommend "kangaroo care," or skin-to skin contact between premature infants and their parents. Recent studies show that this type of care is beneficial to the child, but also improves parental mood and perceptions. Caregivers are hopeful that development of such technology will allow the survival of even younger pre-term infants in the future. This use of an artificial womb is not full ectogenesis as I have defined it, in that the intent here is only to *maintain* fetal life artificially and not also to *initiate* life artificially—a distinction that is morally significant. Full ectogenesis is to be distinguished by the fact that at no point would the gestating fetus be inside of its mother's body.

Apart from the mere scientific intrigue with the ability to artificially incubate embryos into healthy, live infants, there seems to be several general ethical reasons why this AWT might be desirable. Clearly, artificial wombs would be valuable if they could improve the chances to improve premature infant mortality rates or increase the procreative opportunities for individuals who would otherwise be unable to carry a pregnancy to term. But there are more specific reasons why ectogenesis is a gender issue and important to feminists, who are minimally committed to ending the social subordination of women.

Ectogenesis can be examined extensively without reference to gender and is a technology that is likely to render gender less relevant to reproduction or parenting. For this reason alone, artificial wombs have been historically interesting to feminists. But ectogenesis is also relevant to gender because it mimics the biological practice of gestating a child, an ability that currently only women possess, although not all women. Thus, women and men stand to gain and lose from artificial womb technology in different ways and individual women stand to gain or lose differently than other women. To trace these disparate impacts, ectogenesis is a bio-ethical problem requiring analysis sensitive to gender and other socially relevant characteristics. It requires that we consider all parties potentially interested in and affected by ectogenesis. They include not only future merchants and consumers of artificial womb technology, but also women and children whose living bodies will be replaced or subsumed within machinery.

Theories of feminist ethics seem ideally suited for this analytical task. But this analysis is complicated by the plurality of feminist ethics including several different strains not reducible or compatible to one another. Here I consider three main strains of feminist ethics: liberal, radical, and cultural. But it should be noted that there are many other branches of feminist ethics: socialist, post-modern, lesbian, etc., all of which promise to offer new insights into the ethical permissibility of ectogenesis.

2. Liberal Feminism and the Ethics of Artificial Wombs

A liberal feminist analysis of ectogenesis centers on how this technology could increase or decrease the ideals of liberty, equality, and autonomy for women. Liberal feminists believe that female subordination is rooted in customs and legal restraints, which impede women from equally participating in public spheres. Liberal feminism envisions the ideal society as a liberal state in which formal restraints barring women from education, business, and politics are removed, but the basic systemic structures of these institutions remain intact. Ideally, women and men are to be judged as individuals based upon merit, rather than personal and morally arbitrary characteristics like gender.

Like other reproductive technologies such as birth control and abortion, liberal feminists are likely to approve of ectogenesis for at least two reasons. First, artificial wombs could ease the dilemma of having to define equality in terms of the differences or similarities between men and women. Ectogenesis promises to tip the scales in favor of male and female sameness. Since pregnancy and birth are the lynchpins of male/female difference, ectogenesis could create a kind of "sameness" between men and women hitherto unknown. Liberal feminists Susan Moller Okin and James Sterba argue that it is possible and desirable to imagine a society where motherhood is still valued but gender is no longer a socially relevant characteristic.[2] In lasting ways ectogenesis could provide men and women greater reproductive equality by removing the exclusive biological connection between femininity and birth. By divorcing motherhood from female physicality, men could become mothers, easing the maternal burdens of women. There are at least three ways that ectogenesis could allow men to be mothers: a man could be come the immediate and solely human present as a child is removed from the incubator, "mother" could be redefined to refer only to the activity of nurturing, and technology could be developed to allow a man to gestate. In turn, men might become less alienated from birth. Women would no longer have to be negatively impacted by gender-neutral laws and policies that tend to ignore the presently unavoidable biological link between women, pregnancy, and birth.

Second, ectogenesis promises a wider spectrum of reproductive choice for women. Artificial womb technology promises to create freedom in both the negative and positive sense. That is, ectogenesis promises women "freedom from" unwanted pregnancies, and "freedom to" wanted pregnancies prevented by various social and biological circumstances. By way of negative freedom, artificial womb technology promises to free women from both unwanted pregnancies, and unwanted aspects of pregnancy. For instance, supporters of ectogenesis often cite how it could reduce the need for abortion by offering woman a way to avoid pregnancy without having to terminate fetal development.

The freedom from unwanted pregnancy is also likely to enhance women's opportunities in public spheres because of how it would allow them be on the same biological footing as men with regards to birth. No longer would women have to suffer the debilitating effects of pregnancy (e.g. morning sickness, diabetes, and bed rest). Their bodies could be spared the various disfiguring effects that childbirth can bring, both during and after pregnancy. Women could continue to live their normal lives at least nine months longer than they otherwise might were they to incubate a child in their wombs. Pregnancy leave would be unnecessary, except perhaps to allow for bonding with or preparing for the arrival of a developing fetus. Also, women need not be barred from working with dangerous chemicals for fear that their reproductive systems might be damaged.

Ectogenesis offers women positive freedoms in the form of "freedom-to" births that would not otherwise be possible. If artificial womb technology was readily affordable and accessible, they would offer a reproductive alternative to women whose circumstances would normally prevent a natural birth. For example, post-menopausal women, or women at high risk for complications in pregnancy could use ectogenesis to produce a child without a surrogate or birth mother, avoiding potentially messy human and legal relations. Women whose social circumstances make pregnancy less of an option might also benefit from this option. For example, women whose occupations require high physical activity, great public visibility, or high reproductive risks may welcome having ectogenesis as an option to traditional pregnancy. Ectogenesis could become the epitome of family planning, regulating pregnancy and birth rates in a scientific way.

Perhaps the most forceful justification and current motive for the development of AWT for liberal feminists, like most people, is the desire to save fetuses who are miscarried or premature. Liberal feminists are likely to arrive at this point fueled by a desire to prevent the tremendous suffering of women as a result of the loss of a wanted pregnancy, and in this way access to AWT could figure as a very important aspect of women's reproductive health rights in the future. Conceivably, the successful development of AWT could mean that miscarriages would be almost unheard of in the cases of a chromosomally healthy fetus. This use of AWT would be seen as "therapeutic" for both children and mothers.

But liberal feminists also have reason to be concerned about AWT because it could potentially limit or decrease women's freedom, equality, and autonomy. From forced sterilization to chastity belts, history is replete with examples of reproductive technology working to control rather than to liberate women. These technologies also regulated wanted versus unwanted pregnancies but clearly worked against women in design and usage. From a liberal perspective, this is because the technology was a forcible infliction that inhibited women's sexual and reproductive agency, and defined "wanted" and "unwanted" pregnancy in terms other than women's own wishes and desires. Visions of a *Brave New World* aside, it might at first seem a stretch to think that women might someday be forced to reproduce children artificially via machines. But after considering some of the ways that women's behaviors are already regulated with regards to pregnancy, it becomes more plausible that artificial womb technology could reduce women's reproductive liberties, even should women share powerful positions in society.

For example, although it seems doubtful that any woman would be forced to reproduce via ectogenesis, or forbidden from reproducing in natural ways, it is a horrendous possibility should the technology become readily available. For instance, women with drug addictions or who are at high risk to miscarry could be discouraged from the option of natural birth. Women in prison who are pregnant could be forced to deliver their children early. Artificial womb incubation could become an active part of paid sterilization programs.

More drastically, by eradicating the question of fetus viability, ectogenic technology could grant unborn children fuller rights status, and a fetus could be forcibly removed from a woman's womb out of its own interests. Conflicts between the rights of women and fetuses will be heightened greatly as a result of this technology, and norms regarding the starting point of personhood will be even more contentious.

Another likely problem is that ectogenic technology would coerce women's reproductive choices. As Barbara Katz Rothman argues, when reproductive technology opens some doors it tends to close others.[3] Since liberal feminism stops short of reforming basic structures of business, politics, and technological research, it overlooks how public domains are already inhospitable to pregnancy. Were ectogenic technology readily available, a woman's "choice" to compete in these spheres may become even more difficult to balance with the "choice" to carry a pregnancy to term. As a result, many women might feel compelled to choose ectogenesis over natural birth methods in order to maintain their public positions. In turn, the public presence of a pregnant woman might again become a social anomaly. Although it seems far-fetched, it is not implausible that in new ways pregnancy could become perceived as so primitive and disgusting that it feasibly becomes a non-choice. And as this technology is perfected, women's bodies might be pathologized in favor of clinically controllable machinery. Since pregnancy is already a physical condition that is often considered ugly or non-sexual, women who desire to retain their sexual appeal as a social power might perceive little choice but to opt for an artificial pregnancy.

Finally, ectogenesis will very likely be a technology that serves the interests of more powerful members of society, who predominantly continue to be men, retaining some of the current lack of social opportunity for women. There is no guarantee that merely freeing women of their biological connection to pregnancy and birth will ensure that all women can equally participate in education, business, and politics. As scientists develop AWT, women might become reduced to mere wombs and objects of study until the process is perfected, at which time they might become dispensable altogether. Men could "bear" children without anything more in way of female involvement than the donation of eggs. Liberal feminists have supported men taking up the maternal role and believe that should this occur maternity can retain its value. Perhaps allowing men to produce children without the physical presence of a woman will liberate women from certain oppressive bounds of traditional family life, freeing them even more to do non-traditional kinds of work. By distancing women biologically from the process of birth, women's social association with care-giving could be loosened and the concept of motherhood could become a gender neutral activity signified by the conscious activity of nurturing, not a physical process contingent upon biological destiny.

By itself, ectogenesis does not guarantee that this transition will occur. Men could raise children themselves in a very anti-maternal way, and/or pay women to be nannies for children, preserving paternal psychological, legal, and financial control. Obstetrical health care benefits that are already scarce for many women could become more so, if medical and scientific resources are channeled towards ectogenic research, or if a woman with a risky pregnancy choses to gestate her child herself against the advice of her doctors. Without equal gains for women in sciences, medicine, law, and business, ectogenesis is likely to be developed, managed, and accessed by a predominantly male body who will no doubt indivi-dually and collectively profit from such an arrangement. Women who are already socially underprivileged due to race, class, sexual orientation, or nationality, will unlikely to be able to equally exercise a formal right to choose therapeutic use of AWT, but may be compelled to use such technologies should certain social institutions deem them unfit to begin or continue an organic pregnancy.

For liberal feminists the solutions to these problems are to be found in legislation and the use of representational democracy to control the conditions under which AWT is developed and used, as well who is allowed to access it and why. According to this view, once perfected, AWT would be in itself neutral in value. It would be the usage, control, and intent that determines the value of AWT. Liberal feminists could draw upon a feminist version of the harm principle to argue that the ethical and legal permissibility of ectogenesis should track potential harm to women (among others), especially harms associated with diminished agency and choice. For example, liberal feminists might want to make a distinction between (permissible) therapeutic uses of ATW, which would include treatment of miscarried pregnancies, and between more questionable uses of AWT, which might include the incubation of fetuses for convenience sake, for commercial or research purposes, or because a mother is deemed physically or otherwise unfit to carry a pregnancy to term.

Although this principle and distinction remain to be sorted and debated, the successful development of AWT will only kindle constitutional questions about abortion, distributive justice and health care, and personhood. Generally, though, liberal feminism seems to speaks of the ethical permissibility of AWT to the extent that it is an uncoerced choice increasing the reproductive freedom of women, and a resource equally open to all women. It is unclear, however, that at this time or in the future women generally will be able to exercise formal autonomy in this context. And as I shall argue in the next section, it is also unclear that liberal feminism offers an adequate ethical assessment of ectogenesis because it tends to focus on the liberties of women and fetuses independently, overlooking the important relational aspects of pregnancy, birth, and care.

3. Radical Feminism, Cultural Feminism, and the Ethics of Artificial Wombs

The radical strain of feminist philosophy also condones and condemns ectogenesis as a reproductive technology, but for different reasons. Radical feminists are diverse, but what they share is a belief that gender discriminatory laws are merely symptomatic of the true and deeper cause of women's oppression, which they identify as patriarchy built upon biological differences between the sexes. Legislation itself is unlikely to be able to achieve true equality between men and women because social institutions and cultural ideals are rooted in patriarchy, and patriarchy is rooted in fundamental biological differences, namely, differences in muscular strength and sexual reproduction. In other words, before women can rely upon legal channels to achieve sex equality, the biological differences between men and women need to be either altered or accommodated.

Radical feminists are likely to agree that liberal ideals and methods are male biased and not well suited to facilitate the realities of women's biological needs.

However, radical feminists are likely to disagree amongst themselves about the ethics of ectogenesis depending upon how they understand women's biology. Radical feminists who view women's biology as inherently debilitating welcome artificial wombs as technological escape from the natural disadvantages of pregnancy. From this feminist perspective the goal is to change biology. But some radical feminists, such as ecofeminists and cultural feminists, see women's biology as valuable and potentially empowering. They fear that ectogenesis might be a technology that devalues the unique mother-child relationship and bolsters the destruction, commodification, and control of all that is natural. From this feminist perspective the goal is not to change women's biology by relying on AWT, but to revalue women-centered pregnancy and birth. A resistance to mechanized birth is encouraged in favor or organic, holistic, and interpersonal health care. After exploring these two positions further, I will conclude by defending the latter as one that reveals important scientific and cultural problems regarding the development and use of ectogenesis.

Perhaps the most notorious radical feminist who argues in favor of artificial wombs is Shulamith Firestone. Firestone was one of the first feminists to analyze gender inequality on the basis of biology itself, specifically, the biology of procreation. She envisions sex class as springing directly from a biological reality that configures men and women differently, denying them equal privilege.[4] She describes pregnancy as "barbaric" because of its painfulness and brute organic physicality. Firestone argues that reproductive technology has a significant capacity to free women from the oppressive and disgusting aspects of biology, insisting that "we can no longer justify the maintenance of a discriminatory sex class system on the grounds of its origins in Nature. Indeed, for pragmatic reasons ... we *must* get rid of it." Although Firestone explicitly endorses ectogenesis, she observes that women's fears of it are to some extent justified: "in the hands of our current society and under the directions of current scientists (few of whom are female or feminist), any attempted use of technology to 'free' anybody is suspect." But Firestone believes that under the right social conditions, namely full self-determination and economic independence, ectogenesis could be a powerful tool to divorce women from being at "the continual mercy of their biology."

Other radical feminists have identified violence against women as one of the primary vehicles for maintaining patriarchal control. Statistics taken from domestic violence cases show that women are more likely to be battered by their partners while pregnant, and blows inflicted against pregnant women are more likely to be aimed at their abdomens. Less seriously, the visible sign of pregnancy often give others a feeling of entitlement to offer unsolicited advice or to touch a woman's body. Although ectogenesis might not be a solution to all of the basic problems identified by radical feminists, it might be a fair trade-off if it created less opportunity for others to view women's pregnant bodies as personal property, or a justifiable target for violence.

More recently, radical feminists have both supported and rejected Firestone's endorsement of artificial womb technology. For instance, Marge Piercy, in her utopic novel *Women on the Edge of Time*, approvingly imagines a world where children are born in artificial wombs and have three parents, and men can be altered to suckle.[5] But other radical feminists have moved beyond Firestone's idea that pregnancy is inherently oppressive or vicious. Rather, they postulate that the seeming natural disadvantage that women suffer as a result of reproductive biology is largely socially produced. Men as a class have used public and private spheres to demonize and control the meaning of pregnancy and birth. Some of these radical feminists have endorsed "separatism" from men in the form of lesbian and feminist resistance and independence. They call for a revaluation of female-centered motherhood. Lesbian philosophers like Cheshire Calhoun have argued that lesbians should reclaim the ideal of motherhood and family.[6] Again, ectogenesis would seem to facilitate these projects by upsetting the connection between sexual orientation and procreation, and allowing parenthood to be even further removed from heterosexual intercourse. It should be noted, though, that homosexual men stand to benefit from ectogenesis much more so than lesbians, who are as biologically able to gestate children naturally as heterosexual women.

When women's biology is revalued in this way, certain ethical problems with ectogenesis arise. For instance, cultural feminism offers a more disparaging appraisal of ectogenesis, suggesting that what is ethically troubling about artificial wombs is the disintegration of the unique and enigmatic relationship between a mother and child in pregnancy. Cultural feminism is sometimes used to refer to a distinction within radical feminism, and sometimes to the ethics of care, a school of thought that posits that whether by nature or nurture, men and women have developed different sets of values. Both views are likely to reject AWT because it seems yet another step towards not just mechanizing, but demeaning nature, birth, and women's relations to them.

The ethics of care is a perspective associated with the work of Carol Gilligan and others who underscore the relevance of sex to moral reasoning.[7] Care ethicists speculate that the physical aspects of women's reproductive biology can contribute to the development of a relational ethical perspective. Categorizing an ethics of care as a cultural feminism indicates that it is a perspective rooted in symbolically feminine values that are culturally based and empowering to women. An ethics of care takes relationship as an ontological starting point and normative ideal. Fostering reciprocal relationships and nurturing selves through relationship are primary goals. Ideals of care reveal independence to be a potential source of ethical failing when it creates disconnection from the needs of others. The mother-child relationship has been central to the formation of this ideal, which in many ways contrasts starkly with the liberal feminist ideals of liberty, autonomy, and equality, as well as Firestone's ideal of escape from biological motherhood.

The most significant contribution that an ethics of care can make to the deliberation about ectogenesis is to speak to the importance of assessing this technology in terms of relationship and dependency and not just independence and autonomy. For instance, Sara Ruddick, notes that although men and women can both become "mothering-persons," *mothering* must be understood from a female perspective of connection to a child.[8] This position suggests that we cannot make a wholly adequate ethical assessment of artificial womb technology when we only define the interests of women and fetuses apart from one another, since in so doing we ignore the very thing of value which may be potentially lost. Focusing on the mother-child relationship brings to light a number of serious concerns about the development of AWT, some of them scientific, others cultural.

Scientifically, it seems highly risky to progress with the development of AWT when researchers cannot fully identify or duplicate the many physical inter-dynamics between a mother and child in pregnancy. The mother-child gestational relationship is a wholly unique human relation wherein a human is enveloped by another human. Although AWT would theoretically have the capacity to physically gestate a fetus to full term, there is no doubt that this process would differ in significant ways from an organic pregnancy. Most notably, the physical gestational relationship would be drastically altered. The use of AWT would be controversial even if it was relatively perfected with no chance for error, but the development of full term AWT is even more controversial because it requires at some point that scientists move beyond "therapeutic" AWT to the incubation of children fertilized in test tubes and a complete physical separation of a mother and fetus for the entire gestational period. Although all technologies have their pioneer human subjects and the first of these to be artificially incubated are likely to be fetuses who will die without it, part of the problem is that we do not yet have a full understanding of what gestational relationship involves, or how it correlates to post-partum health of both mother and child. Scientists are just beginning to conceptualize the myriad levels on which mothers and unborn children interact, and these processes are not yet entirely identified, much less understood.

For instance, scientists know that infants receive immunities from their mother's bodies in the womb and while breast-feeding. They also recognize that the immunity process and breast milk stimulation are just two examples of how mothers and children interact on both physical and psychological levels. For example, breast milk is often stimulated by the cry of a baby, and the composition of breast milk varies depending upon how long a mother nurses, her food choices and state of mind, as well as the specific antibodies in her system. But scientists do not yet understand, and cannot simulate, this immunity process completely. They have not been able to identify, much less duplicate, all of the components of breast milk, which transfer immunities and nutrients from mother to child. The transference of immunities during the process of pregnancy via amniotic fluid and the umbilical cord is even less understood, but it is reasonable to presume that this, too, is not merely a mechanical process that can be replicated without removing an essential human factor from the process of birth. Without more knowledge, ectogenic babies would not receive immunities from their mothers during pregnancy, and possibly not after birth either since breast milk is only stimulated in some women by the actual experience of pregnancy. Even if at some point scientists may be able to replicate this physical process to a degree adequate to sustain fetal health, just as they have developed "formula" nutritionally adequate to replace breast-milk, we can only speculate about the existence of other such processes, and about how much of the human organic birth connection can be shaved away without damage to both mother and fetus.

Recent studies show that during pregnancy the bodies of mother and child interact with one another not only in a one-way transference of nutrients from mother to child, but in a two-way interaction that is dynamic and responsive. Researchers looking for the cause of an immune disorder in some women have traced it back to the presence of Y chromosomes in the cellular make up of these women as a result of previously gestating and giving birth to male infants. The presence of Y-chromosomes indicates that fetuses are not just passive recipients of nutrients, but on the cellular and physical level they give in return to the bodies of their mothers.

Another example of a mother-child interaction is the better known Rh negative factor that causes women with Rh-negative blood to create antibodies against the incompatible blood cells of a gestating child. Although these are both examples of mother-child interactions that are potentially harmful, they intimate the presence of other interactions that have more positive implications and are less noticeable because nothing goes wrong.

What is significant about these findings is that the model of the womb as the fetal container, or the placenta as a one-way supplier of nutrients and remover of waste is inadequate, because pregnancy is instead an exchange of growth and development. In this way AWT has medical and scientific implications for the health of women as well as of children.

What is even less clear is the emotional and psychological relationships that might occur as a result of a child developing inside of a mother's womb. Studies conducted in the last two decades indicate that when mothers use sound and touch to stimulate a child in utero this improves the subsequent development of the child after birth.[9] Newborn babies are able to distinguish their mother's voice from those of strangers and to recognize music that was regularly played to them while they were gestating. If it makes sense to believe that playing Mozart is enriching to an unborn child, it is certainly not unreasonable to suppose that newborns are developing important relational capacities as a result of hearing their mother's voices and rhythmic heartbeats. The experience of being enveloped in flesh may be a precondition for human affection and intimacy that contributes to a need for human contact.

Both animal studies and observations of children in orphanages have shown that maternal deprivation immediately after birth can severely impact a child's ability to communicate and relate. It may be that relational deprivation prior to birth could have similar negative effects. Also, while it is possible that a full gestational relationship could be simulated through the use of audio tape, visitation, or the male-bowel-pregnancy, it is unknown whether these replacements could fully duplicate the physical, psychological, and emotional interactions of the female organic pregnancy. Let us try to imagine the most fully realizable simulation of an artificial womb possible. This virtual womb is complete with not only with nutrients and metal rods, but also sounds, movements, and perhaps even simulated tissue, hormones, and fluid filled placenta. Voices of future family members are piped in as well other sounds of the womb. The umbilical cord is replaced by finely crafted tubing which somehow delivers the proper neonatal formula and rids the fetal body of waste. The question still remains whether we can successfully imitate the dynamic and unpredictable variables of these components as they come together in the body of a living woman subject to a emotional, social, and intellectual life. Certainly "mothers" could visit their incubating babies to speak to them and otherwise interact, but would this interaction be of the same kind and degree that evolves in an organic pregnancy?

We do not know how much a fetal body and mind is impacted by being inside a woman's body, or how a woman's body and mind is impacted as a result of pregnancy. Minimally, however, this analysis suggests that ectogenic research and development should strive as much as possible to simulate other features of organic gestation besides mere minimal physical components of nutrition and waste removal. But this task poses great epistemological challenges since we cannot access the perceptual life of a fetus, and it is an open philosophical and scientific question about how human development is affected by experiences in the womb. The development of AWT is already being conducted on animals, but the observation of animals cannot entirely reveal the psychological and social aspects of human life (and this use of animals is ethically questionable from this feminist point of view for many of the same reasons). If Thomas Nagel is correct to say that we cannot know what it is like to be a bat, similarly we cannot know what it is like to be a fetus: we can only observe the physical unfolding of it. Absent this perspectival access, women who have experienced pregnancy may be able to fill in part of the picture from their perspective. This perspective would always be relational, but it would always be a one-way perspective of this relationship, and thus incomplete. We seem unable to fully anticipate the potential damage to a fetus incubated artificially.

One apparent objection to this line of argument is that ectogenesis would be no different than fatherhood or adoption and in some ways this is true. Most fathers, as well as women who adopt do not directly experience the gestational relationship, yet are able to bond readily with their children. But what is mistaken about this analogy is that it loses sight of the gestational relationship between a child and *someone*, which may serve as an important precondition of bonding, *for the child*, and in turn for the parent. Ectogenesis as I have defined it is unprecedented in that it creates a human being who has no "birth mother" in the usual sense, and it is uncertain how this will affect the relational potential of a child. As Nel Noddings has suggested, the capacity for receptivity and response in a child can serve as an important motivational pay-off for a caregiver.[10] If children who are gestated artificially miss out on stimuli that are pre-conditions for human relationship this could have tremendous social and psychological implications.

But even if it turns out that there is no discernable difference in the physical and emotional health of children born artificially from those born organically, this does not mean that AWT ceases to be medically and scientifically questionable given the relationship between mothers and children. Pregnancy and lactation are known to have certain health benefits for women, in that pregnancy and breastfeeding have been linked to decreased risk of breast cancer in women.

The physical relationship of pregnancy can also impact the emotional and psychological development of women who experience it. Pregnant women can begin shifting into a kind of relational frame-of-mind where they have a constant sense of being with another, of being a "we" rather than an "I." Pregnant women might talk or sing to their unborn child as a result of a kick or a turn. Contractions in pregnant women, and milk flow in nursing mothers can be stimulated by physical and emotional sensations.

While not all pregnant women develop such a relational psychology when pregnant or after giving birth, this should not lead us to ignore the way that organic pregnancy *can* foster a relationship that goes beyond the mere physical aspects of gestation. Would the use of AWT lead to an increased biological, emotional, and physical distance between mothers and children, and hence to society in general?

This leads to the second objection to ectogenesis posed by radical, cultural, and environmental feminisms. A common thread between these feminist perspectives is a reverence for motherhood and a commitment to counteracting cultural forces that work against women as mothers. Although the activities and meanings associated with motherhood are as culturally diverse as women themselves, motherhood is a universal and mythic theme directly linked to the social status of actual women in actual societies. These perspectives recognize that although motherhood is a site of potential oppression for women, it is also a site of potential empowerment, and ectogenesis is to be assessed in terms of how it will increase or decrease this power. They also recognize that there is direct correlation between the cultural value of motherhood and the lives of real women and children.

In some cultures giving birth is one of the most significant ways in which woman can achieve social status because it is hard not to recognize pregnancy and birth as acts of trial, commitment, and accomplishment. Although it is sometimes hard to tell in our society, pregnancy, birth, and motherhood can be inherently empowering for women in many ways. Radical feminists see the ability to bring forth life as a capacity that men have long envied and tried to control. Much radical feminist literature has been committed to uncovering a cultural fear of maternal power, and to demonstrating that beneath a shallow reverence for mothers are patriarchal social frameworks that undermine and malign maternal authority. Naming is just one way this occurs in patriarchal societies. Surnames, or "Sir names" indicate patrilineage and imply the historical precedent of seeing children as the property of fathers, not mothers. Many common surnames convey the primacy of the father and the male offspring: "Peter-son," "John-son," "Richard-son," etc. Likewise, in western art and religion, mothers (when they are present at all) are often portrayed as neglectful, manipulative, crazy, pathetically ineffective, or virtuously powerless, and rarely do they serve as cultural heroes or divinities.[11] In practice, motherhood and domestic work are unpaid and considered menial, putting mothers in positions of dependency and inferiority in relation to both husbands and the state. Ectogenesis is an objectionable technology from this perspective because of how it seems to continue these trends by demeaning the cultural significance of female biology and nature, and by reducing the power of women as mothers.

Ectogenesis is problematic from these feminist perspectives because of how it could further demean women's biology as part of a general campaign against nature. Ecofeminists contend that feminine biology has been considered culturally coextensive with nature (e.g. "Mother Nature") and that both have been portrayed as wild, irrational, and in need of being mastered. Western culture makes meaning of the world by relying upon dualisms that facilitate patriarchal dominance not only by portraying certain concepts as opposite in meaning but also in value. Femininity and masculinity, body and reason, nature and culture—these dualisms often correspond to evil and good, the savage and the civilized. As Val Plumwood suggests, to be defined as nature (as opposed to reason) is to be defined as a passive non-agent and non-subject. It is to be defined as an environment, i.e., as a set of invisible background conditions against which is foregrounded the achievements of reason or culture, a resource empty of its own purpose or meanings and hence available to be annexed for the purposes identified by reason.[12] This general critique can be used to further diagnose some of the ways in which ectogenesis might serve to demean women's biology and decrease the power of women.

Ectogenesis treats women's reproductive biology in the way described by Plumwood by substituting a female body with a machine void of consciousness, and subject to man-made controls and purposes. The idea that the mother-child relation in pregnancy could even begin to be adequately simulated by a machine implies a problematic Cartesian model of mind and matter that portrays pregnancy as a mere mechanical process. AWT is a technology that objectifies and produces only a crude facsimile of a woman's body. AWT objectifies women's bodies in a very literal sense by reducing a mother to a body part, the womb, only to simulate this body part by constructing a disembodied, non-rational, mechanical object.

AWT also shows a remarkable disrespect for nature and the wisdom of the body—a concept that is even difficult to grasp using Western medical models. The body of a woman often knows automatically how to nurture and gestate a child even when women themselves and the experts are ignorant. It can internally alter itself and adapt to a variety of challenging circumstances, identifying and filtering out environmental toxins for the growing child. Doctors are finding, for example, that women suffering from breast cancer can receive chemotherapy while pregnant because their bodies somehow are able to filter out or neutralize these toxic chemicals for their babies.[13] Other things known about pregnancy today show that women's bodies interact with their environments. For example, women's bodies track the cycles of the moon and the menstrual cycles of women living together will gradually shift to coincide. The earlier onset of menarche of girls in the U.S. is theorized to be due to increased sexual stimuli and a diet including bovine hormones. A range of recent studies suggests that eating fish while pregnant and lactating leads to the overall mental health of mother and child.[14] All of this suggests that women's bodies are not solely mechanical and that a machine is not an adequate simulation of a mother.

Ectogenesis is also the ultimate example of how nature is being increasingly replaced by machines that run off nonrenewable resources, requiring further natural destruction to fuel the technology. Therapeutic use of AWT to save premature infants might seem urgent enough to warrant such uses of technology, but there are real ecological questions about the need for ectogenesis to supplement natural births. Although it seems like the makings of a crude joke, a startlingly practical concern that emerges from this line of thought is what might happen should fetuses gestating artificially within electric machines for some reason get caught in a power outage without the benefit of backup generators. There are relevant concerns about population growth and the need for AWT when there is a plethora of unwanted children available for adoption. An argument can be made that the use of AWT will reduce the living conditions of some women and children in order to bring about the birth of the globally elite.

But ectogenesis is also disturbing because of how it could further strip women of immediate maternal power. Cultural and radical feminists have traced the historical ways in which pregnancy and birth have become increasingly mediated by "experts" and social authorities who have traditionally been men. Even though today these mediators are more likely to include women, they still tend to operate within systems and institutions that are coded as masculine. There is no reason to think that ectogenesis will not follow this trend. Ectogenesis would mean that a mother gives up a direct measure of power over her offspring in virtue of the fact that her child does not grow inside of her body. Removed to an incubator, a child is more subject to the decisions and opinions of others, as well as being more vulnerable to kidnapping, tampering, and neglect. It is certainly a mistake to portray all mothers as unwavering protectors of children, but it cannot be denied that mothers generally tend to be their children's fiercest guardians. A frightening loss of power for mothers and future children with regards to AWT is the ease with which a child could be born without the presence of a woman who is most likely to have a physical and psychological bond to her. Pedophiles, religious cults, or unscrupulous military systems could certainly thrive even more than they already do from the use of ectogenesis. The numbers and value of living women might even decrease, since sex-selective birth practices that lead to dispro-portionate numbers of boys would no longer necessarily have dire reproductive results. While liberal feminism has difficulty asserting the rights of potential persons, a feminist ethic that emphasizes relationship allows us to consider our relationship and obligations to future children who might be born through ectogenesis without mothers.

Liberal and radical feminists can agree that a high degree of reverence for motherhood can sometimes be a vehicle for controlling women and that it is important for women to be able to freely determine the cultural value of motherhood. But there are important differences in the way that liberal and radical feminists might assess ectogenesis in this context. For example, in industrial capitalist societies like the United States, the activities associated with mother-hood are increasingly provided by for-profit businesses, and machines perform many tasks that were once performed by women themselves. Liberal feminists generally herald the above trends as progress, but radical and cultural feminists are more cautious in their approval. From their perspective, ectogenesis can be seen as another huge step in the direction of making mothers more like traditional fathers—physically and emotionally distant from children and the activities of care.

Ectogenesis promises to reconfigure the cultural meaning of terms like "birth" and "mother" in alarming ways. For example, what would it mean for a child gestated artificially to be "born"? Would it refer to when she was a full term infant, to the precise moment when she was disconnected and removed from machinery, or to when she was handed over to the custody of a caregiver? The celebration of the birthday of an artificially gestated child would herald a different kind of significance, as would the notion of a "mother." Many feminists working within the care ethic have moved towards defining "mother" as someone who performs the activity of nurturing a child, but for many people, the term "mother" inherently connotes a woman who is pregnant and gives birth. Even the distinction between "birth mothers" and "adoptive mothers" would dissolve for children born from ectogenesis, since they would have no actual "birth mother" but only a "genetic mother" who has merely made the biological contribution of an egg. If ectogenesis was to be combined with other reproductive technologies, this donation conceivably could even come from fetal tissue or a cloned cell. Since the word "father" has been traditionally more associated with the distanced donation of biological material, AWT has the real potential to further shift the cultural meaning of motherhood to a more masculine model.

Furthermore, unlike liberal feminists who would endorse AWT if it were desired by women without questioning the reasons why women might so desire it, radical and cultural feminists posit that women sometimes suffer from "false consciousness." That is, women can have desires produced by coercive socialization that works against their true interests. They note, for example, that women often desire to conform to beauty standards in order to make their bodies sexually desirable to men even when this means damaging their own health and mobility. Current beauty standards for women emphasize extreme thinness, a trend that some radical feminists attribute in part to a latent anti-maternalism. Although the importance of relationship in cultural feminism commits it to acknowledging the ways in which AWT might nurture relations by saving premature infants, radical feminism reveals that there are other motivations fueling ectogenesis stemming from scientific and cultural atmospheres that pathologize pregnancy, birth, and female physiology. Radical and cultural feminists resist social trends that equate the empowerment of women with the suppression of all things coded as feminine, include female biology and nature. They are likely to join with ecofeminists in protesting ectogenesis as part of a broad move to control nature and replace it with man-made machinery. The perception of pregnancy as a disfiguring disability, pregnant women as potential contaminators of fetuses, and birth as "barbaric," fosters an environment that makes AWT seem attractive because it promises to be more safe, sterile, and pain free than "natural" childbirth. Thus, even if ectogenesis becomes a reproductive choice for women, radical feminists are likely to argue that there are good reasons why women should resist this choice.

Can anything be said in favor of the brute physicality of pregnancy and birth against ectogenesis? Although few women are likely to praise all of the physical aspects of pregnancy, many are likely to see it as worthwhile and sometimes even pleasurable. The physical changes of pregnancy can help prepare women psychologically for motherhood and childcare. A changing body is an obvious external sign to a woman and others that something life-altering is about to occur. Even labor pains can vividly contribute to a woman feeling that a child is something to be worked for and valued. Contributing first hand to the physical growth and birth of children can create a physical sense of responsibility and entitlement with regards to those children that is recognized by self and others. The experience of pregnancy and birth gives women a kind of natural authority over their children that is recognized both formally and informally. Courts in the U.S. give prima facie preference to birth mothers in custody battles acknowledging the importance of the physical, biological aspects of pregnancy and birth. A mother of a child produced by ectogenesis would be on the same biological footing as the father in a custody case. In this way, women as a class could see a loss of legal power. Informally, the experience of pregnancy and birth can give a mother leverage within her family. For example, although it is not always as immediately effective as she might wish, a mother might remind her children of her struggles in childbirth as a way of establishing her authority.

Of course, the availability of AWT is unlikely to mean that most women couldn't have a "natural" pregnancy should they choose, but this doesn't mean that the cultural meaning and attitudes towards natural pregnancy would not shift. One such change might be that natural birth loses some of its power to awe and is seen instead as something "old fashioned" and primitive. Even some feminists have agreed with the idea that pregnancy and mothering is largely a mechanical and thoughtless process. As Charlotte Perkins Gilman put it: even a bird will sit on a stone if it looks like an egg. The conceptualization of pregnancy as a mere mechanical process that a machine could and should duplicate, only reinforces the idea that women contribute nothing especially intellectual or unique to the process of human gestation. Women who did choose to have natural births when AWT was available and encouraged might have their pain and discomfort viewed as a deserved outcome of a foolish decision. Feasibly, ectogenesis and AWT could even become seen as part of "pain management" for women.

Finally, if it is true that pregnancy can serve to augment empathetic capacities of women (and children), then it is possible that increased reliance on ectogenesis could broadly contribute to increased social alienation and antagonism. Pregnancy hormones often make women more emotionally sensitive, and the physical bulk of pregnancy can remind women of what it is like to be physically dependent in varying degrees. The familiarity that a newborn shows to its mother's body cannot be underestimated in its power to shape the human psyche. It is unknown whether an artificially incubated child would develop a similar affinity to the machine that gestated him. But regular use of ectogenesis to produce children would result in fewer women and children experiencing the bond of pregnancy, which would directly translate into an immediate reconfiguration of the intimate relational aspects of family and society. The larger implications of ectogenesis remains to be seen, but it seems reasonable to speculate that using AWT beyond the "therapeutic" treatment of premature infants will make human relations even more alienated and self-centered.

4. Conclusion

I have shown that liberal and radical feminists are likely to both support and reject the ethical permissibility of ectogenesis. Liberal feminism highlights the liberating potential of ectogenesis provided that women are able to equally shape and access this technology. Radical feminism suggests that ectogenesis could open up positive new ways of configuring male and female relationship by altering the biology of sex difference. However, an ethics of care drawing from radical, cultural, and ecofeminism reveals potential downsides of artificial wombs that must be weighed against the more promising aspects of this technology for women. Specifically, there is a real question about whether scientists will ever be able to fully duplicate the complex and myriad interrelations between mother and fetus in the gestational relationship. Ectogenesis also has the potential to shift the cultural meaning of pregnancy, birth, and motherhood, further alienating humanity from nature.

My argument suggests that the assessment of ectogenesis is incomplete when considered only from moral and scientific frameworks that subdivide the interests and relationships of pregnant women and unborn children. It also suggests that if research and development of AWT should proceed, it should not do so without consideration of the developmental value of gestational relationship. It should avoid the objectification of women and fetuses as mere entities of study and include women's subjective understandings about the value of organic pregnancy and birth.

Ultimately, feminists have reason to entertain moral approval only for "therapeutic" uses of AWT that aim at saving spontaneously miscarried fetuses, and to stand against the development and use of full ectogenesis on the principle that it is inherently demeaning and disempowering to women as biological mothers. Both culturally and as individuals, mothers and children alike may suffer real loss the day that it finally can be said that the first human child has been "of machine born."

NOTES

1. Reported on ABC-Chicago "Healthbeat" (23 September 2002).

2. Susan Moller Okin, *Justice, Gender, and the Family* (New York: Basic Books, 1989), p. 178. James Sterba, "Feminist Justice and Sexual Harassment," *Journal of Social Philosophy* 27 (1996), pp. 103–122.

3. Barbara Katz Rothman, "The Meanings of Choice in Reproductive Technology," in *Test-tube Women: What Future for Motherhood*, ed. Rita Arditti, Renate Duelli Klein, and Shelley Minden (London: Pandora Press, 1984), pp. 23–33.

4. Shulamith Firestone, *The Dialectic of Sex: The Case for Feminist Revolution* (New York: William Morrow and Co., 1970), pp. 232–236.

5. Marge Piercy, *Women on the Edge of Time* (New York: Ballentine Books, 1983).

6. Cheshire Calhoun, *Feminism, Family, and the Politics of the Closet: Gay and Lesbian Displacement* (New York: Oxford University Press, 1983).

7. Carol Gilligan, *In a Different Voice: Psychological Theory and Women's Development* (Cambridge, Mass.: Harvard University Press, 1982).

8. Sara Ruddick, *Maternal Thinking* (Boston: Beacon Press, 1989), p. 15.

9. Beatriz Manrique, *Pregnancy and Early Stimulation of Babies* (Caracas, Venezuela: State Department for Intelligence Development, 2000).

10. Nel Noddings, *Caring* (Berkeley: University of California Press, 1984).

11. Kathryn Allen Rabuzzi, *Motherself: A Mythic Analysis of Motherhood* (Bloomington: Indiana University Press, 1988), pp. 63–64.

12. Val Plumwood, *Feminism and the Mastery of Nature* (London and New York: Routledge, 1993), p. 4.

13. Reported on NBC's *Dateline* (4 August 2003).

14. Laird Harrison, "Eating Fish during Pregnancy and Lactation may Benefit Mother and Child," *Psychology Today* 34 (November-December 2001), p. 26.

Nine

ECTOGENESIS: LIBERATION, TECHNOLOGICAL TYRANNY, OR JUST MORE OF THE SAME?

Joan Woolfrey

In what seems like a world far away and long ago, Shulamith Firestone published one of the works that would become a treatise for a new generation. In *The Dialectic of Sex*, Firestone argued, among other things, that the oppression of women would not be eradicated until women no longer functioned as the sole means of reproducing the species.[1] Until an alternative to the traditional means of reproduction was developed via technological advance, and until women in general, and feminists in particular, had more control over that technology, this world would continue to produce suffering by markedly ignoring issues of gender injustice. Firestone maintained that, until such a time as reproduction no longer depended upon women's bodies, women would be encouraged to be, and would see themselves as rightly, defined by their reproductive biology. Women would thus continue to be enslaved to their reproductive function. We are on the verge of a technological advance which bears directly on Firestone's predictions: artificial womb technology or "ectogenesis." Research at the University of Tokyo, Juntendo University in Tokyo, Leeds University in England, and Cornell and Temple Universities in this country, and elsewhere progresses towards the development of artificial environments for fetuses. Predictions range from 10 to 30 years before the work will be ready for human use.

It seems appropriate to ponder ethical issues raised by Firestone in 1970 in light of the realities of today; to examine some of the ethical questions technological access to ectogenesis triggers for our society through Firestone's lens. Most prominent amongst the observations I make is a recognition that such technology has little potential for improving the status of women at this time in this society's history. This would be no surprise to Firestone, who contended that the radical re-structuring of society would need to accompany any such technological advance for it to produce its liberating effects. Rather than seeing artificial womb technology as the necessary and sufficient condition for liberation, it would be consistent with Firestone's work to see such technology as the final rung on the liberation ladder—a necessary but by no means sufficient condition for equality. Within society's current construction, there is reason to believe that increasing the options for circumventing infertility or the lack of a partner will only perpetuate the overemphasis placed on the reproductive capacities of women.

That this society encourages such a trend is a topic that has been dealt with by a number of scholars including Janice Raymond, Gena Corea, and Mary O'Brien.[2] I will not be reviewing that literature here.

1. Ectogenesis and Women's Value

In my view, ectogenesis, coming of age in the current environment, will only serve to perpetuate an over-emphasis on women's reproductive functions, a tendency that seems inevitable considering the intended use of the first generation of this impending technology. The fruits of the labor of researchers in the U.S. and in Japan in the area of ectogenesis aim to benefit extremely low birthweight babies. Research meant to make artificial wombs a reality exists in order to increase the chances of survival for the smallest of premature infants and for fetuses with conditions that would benefit from closer monitoring than a womb can provide. Such technology grants an option to parents who would otherwise lose their infants or be faced with the potential for the massive health problems often associated with extremely premature birth.

In addition, while potentially increasing survival rates for the most vulnerable pregnancies—and, no doubt, being a great source of relief for anxious and frightened parents—this technology is also poised, I argue, to encourage the perpetuation of the notion that motherhood is women's most important function. That motherhood should not be women's most important function will not be fully argued here. I hope it is sufficient to state that human beings living to their full potential cannot be compartmentalized in such a narrow fashion. That society currently sends that message will not be fully argued here either. For those who need evidence, the personal testimony of any number of voluntarily or involuntarily childless women in this society may be sufficient.

Support for this view on the effect of the artificial womb on women can be found in the incentives that exist for this kind of research. (1) The funding is available. The money can be and has been found to support this kind of research. (2) Researchers exist who see value in embarking on research in this direction, and are intrigued by the problems it presents. (3) There are often desperate and no doubt genuine demands by women, by couples, for techniques that will help them successfully circumvent problem pregnancies and infertility. Once this technology is available, there will be heart-wrenching pleas for it—and a market that thrives on supply and demand. (4) The institutional environment of academia can, does, and will, enthusiastically encourage such pursuits.

I am not suggesting that such incentives, taken individually, warrant criticism. I am suggesting, however, that when we consider these individual elements in light of other societal issues, we find that such factors combine to reinforce the oppressive structures in our society which serve to converge into a focus on the reproductive capacities of women to the exclusion of all else that they can be. Christine Overall, for one, discusses the repercussions of living in what she calls a pro-natalist, but anti-child, society.[3] Support for her view comes, in part, from attending to the amount and variety of resources which this society expends on matters relevant to the first few weeks of life. After those first few months, the attention wanes. On average, a child born prior to 26 weeks gestation stays in the hospital for four months and costs $250,000.[4] What this society spends on the prevention of child abuse per potentially abused child is difficult to estimate, but several state studies suggest the amount is miniscule in comparison.[5] We, as a society, do not appear to have the same compelling interest in saving a child from sexual abuse or poverty as we do in ensuring the survival of a 23 week old fetus born prematurely. The further removed from birth, the less willing our society seems to be to allocate resources. No insurance industry has arisen, for instance, around the probability of single parenthood following divorce—one of the contributing causes of childhood poverty. The federal poverty level and the minimum wage meet continuing criticism for inadequately providing for our nation's children.

In some respects, it is no surprise that science and technology researchers focus their energies on the neo-natal phase of life. That phase represents challenges particularly suited to technological and scientific enterprises, as currently conceived. Poverty and abuse cannot compete. The subject matter of those problems is not as sexy. Society's attention wanes after infancy at least partly because science has not understood itself as having a role to play in what has been viewed as allocation of resources and social services problems. And, the social work and public and mental health fields, which traditionally focus on tending to the needs of the most vulnerable members of our society, do not carry the same prestige as science. Problems related to poverty and abuse do not seem to appeal to those who pursue the complex questions at the beginning of life. At any rate, my point here is that what is interesting about the research currently being done in the direction of ectogenesis is linked to the kinds of values which science, and society at large, recognizes. Mastering life's forces, solving the puzzles of the origins of life, and gaining technological control over the reproduction process are examples of the sorts of research that can bring prestige and renown to researchers in the current scientific environment. Questions not perceived to contain the same provocative, profound, glamorous results will be less likely to attract the same quality of researcher, the same number of research dollars.

Research into the problems of poverty and abuse could become as prestigious as cancer research or experimental surgical procedures *in utero* or on neonates. Work in other disciplines could eventually be seen as just as noble, just as worthy of financial support, just as important to institutions that provide the facilities for research, and, thus, just as appealing to the cream of the crop of our academic institutions. Our society would have to undergo seismic transformations in order for the ground to be laid for such an emphasis, however.

Women's reproductive functions receive inordinate attention because science and technology are particularly well-suited to contribute in this area, on a *psychological,* as well as a technological, level. While inherent differences exist which may explain, if not justify, the scientific focus on reproduction rather than poverty, such a distinction does not explain why reproduction appears to be so much more attractive than, for example, the importance of other physiological differences between men and women such as metabolism or bone structure. Intuitively, it may not seem difficult to find explanations for why reproduction fascinates so much more readily, than, say, the origins of a bleeding ulcer. The creation of life has intrigued and mystified human beings for eons. To examine that fascination closely, however, leads us to an account of the myriad ways in which society continues to overemphasize women's biological capacities.

There is not space here to explore the origins and ramifications of that fascination; for now, it will have to be sufficient to take notice of the several billion dollar-a-year reproductive technologies industry that has grown up around the demand by women and couples for ways to circumvent infertility, and the eagerness of researchers and infertility clinic entrepreneurs to find more and more efficient and predictable ways for satisfying the consumers of these services. These are expressions of the demands of a society—at least its more vocal and visible segments—heavily focused on reproduction.

British sociologist Sarah Franklin has commented, with irony, on this overemphasis on female reproduction and its immediate aftermath. "[T]housands of comparatively privileged women worldwide" go to startling technological and financial lengths in the pursuit of parenthood while "many times as many other women" lack access to the simplest contraceptives.[6] If women were valued more for their human potential outside of their reproductive functions, it can be argued, this contrast would not be so stark. I see both aspects of this irony as support for the overemphasis on motherhood. (1) Worldwide, societies encourage women to see themselves primarily as mothers. Lack of access to contraceptives can more easily be dismissed as unimportant due to that perceived inevitability. (2) Women or couples who cannot reproduce naturally and have the resources to pursue fertility treatments, often do so with an astonishing vehemence and all-encompassing focus.

Pursuit of motherhood becomes the central focus of life for many, as Elizabeth Bartholet admits from personal experience in her article "In Vitro Fertilization: The Construction of Infertility and Parenting."[7] It can become such a single-minded pursuit that all other aspects of one's life will suffer. In Bartholet's words, "[t]he treatment process is so intensive that it is almost impossible to get through it *without* focusing most of your life energies on the attempt to become pregnant."[8] If infertility were not viewed as a disease in this society, in need of medical intervention, and if women were understood—and understood themselves—to be quite complete and valuable human beings whether or not they give birth, the spotlight might not shine quite so brightly on the development of additional technological means for circumventing infertility and problem pregnancies. If we viewed women as consistently and importantly valuable outside of their reproductive functions, we as a society might find it more worthwhile to encourage the spread of contraceptive information, and of responsible sex practices, to a greater degree than we currently do. If we cared more about the human potential of all, we would likely be doing more to encourage the development of the wide range of skills and abilities of girls and women, and to ensure that the potential for such pursuits remains intact, amongst those members of society already in existence.

In light of what I have said so far, the greatest ethical concerns regarding reproductive technologies generally, and the future of ectogenesis particularly, appear to be largely two-fold. First, in a world with limited resources, focusing large amounts of money and time in an area which will benefit relatively few is difficult to justify, when there are more severe problems perhaps *more* deserving of our time and attention, e.g., poverty and abuse. And, second, encouraging the reproductive pursuits of females to the extent that it detracts from all else that they can be is an unjust feature of our society, especially when that encouragement speaks to the very core of one's self-concept, and thus self-worth. But the concerns expressed thus far are not aimed solely at what is new about ectogenesis. I would like to direct my attentions for the remainder of this paper to ethical questions raised by ectogenesis in particular.

2. Ethical Issues Specific to Ectogenesis

Ectogenesis, as currently envisioned, is meant to be a haven for fetuses born too soon or so ill that close monitoring of this type will raise their chances of survival. It is a technology meant to be an aid in successful functioning of particularly difficult reproductive processes. It encourages an emphasis on women's reproductive functions in that it is meant to be a replacement for the natural progression of a pregnancy when such a process fails or appears inadequate. Women in a position to benefit from such technology will also bear the psychological burden of being possessed of a body perceived by many, themselves included, to have failed. An argument could be made that to embark on a technology that will create such burdens without also addressing and attempting to alleviate these kinds of negative consequences is to engage in irresponsible science. This is an aspect of ectogenesis that should not be ignored. Similarly, building scores of nuclear plants without a clear plan for permanently disposing of the deadly waste, it can be argued, is irresponsible science and legislating. To take an action, aware of the potential for negative consequences, without taking all reasonable precautions is morally irresponsible. I will not anchor this familiar argument in the interest of space constraints.

But, let's wander even further down the research road. In theory, ectogenesis *could* eventually become an alternative method of reproduction, altogether eliminating the necessity for women to carry a pregnancy to term and give birth. Such an option, Shulamith Firestone claimed, was one step in bringing women closer to freedom from the constricting view society encourages: that women should be, first and foremost, baby-makers.

I wish to test the proposal by Firestone that such technology could be liberating. Since the liberation demanded is from an unjust social structure, such liberation is an ethical imperative in Firestone's work. How would society have to change in order for technological advances of this kind to have the effect she predicted—of freeing women from being undervalued and of being constricted because of gender by various interrelated barriers in our society? "Extrauterine fetal incubation" (another term for ectogenesis), as currently envisioned, will likely save more preemies from death and disability than can be done currently.

The question being raised here is: Could ectogenesis (would it) do more? If ectogenesis becomes a conveniently available option to a woman's uterus, might it release women from the bonds of reproduction and child-rearing and thus free them from being undervalued by being subordinated to those particular tasks? Would we be closer to a truly egalitarian society if reproduction did not rely on a woman's biological functions?

My view parallels Franklin's work. She argues that rather than "challenge the nuclear family, ... enable women to be less defined by their reproductive capacity, ... develop more feminist definitions of biology, or ... dissolve the patriarchal structures of society," ectogenesis, as a future segment of the reproductive technologies industry, is bound to increase the desperation of infertile women, encourage the views that families are incomplete without children and women are deficient unless they are mothers, and exploit the "right" of (at least) heterosexual couples to reproduce.[9] The following discussion elaborates on this position.

3. Ectogenesis as Medical Necessity

If it is a matter of emergency—of a pregnancy that will not continue in a woman's body and a fetus thus endangered—and the potential exists for the fetus to be saved by use of an artificial womb, there seems to be nothing outside of the concerns already mentioned (namely, resource allocation, and the psychological burdens of a body that has "failed") that would give us ethical pause.

4. Ectogenesis as Pregnancy Option

If this technology, once refined, were available to anyone who would choose it, as an alternative to a pregnancy carried inside a woman's body, what ethical concerns, if any, would be raised? Setting aside Firestone for a moment, is there anything unethical about choosing not to carry a pregnancy to term inside one's own body, a process one nevertheless wishes to have occur? However bizarre or unnatural one might initially think such a suggestion is, neither reaction specifically comments on the ethics of the matter.[10] To voluntarily forego the connection, the relationship, that can develop between a mother and her fetus is to instead rely on the kind of relationship that a father currently can have. If genuine caring exists, being inside or outside a human body during early development seems irrelevant. If genuine connection does *not* exist, being inside or outside a human body again seems unlikely to make any difference. To choose to have a child, but be unwilling or unable to carry it is not new. We as a society have been grappling with issues related to the modern surrogacy industry for decades now. Most concerns raised around that issue relate specifically to the surrogate. Are we treating the woman as a means by renting her womb to have our babies? Are we objectifying, instrumentalizing, or commodifying human beings who are willing to bear children for others? Whatever our answers to these questions, they will be irrelevant to ectogenesis, as there is no human surrogate in this case.

A woman who chooses ectogenesis in order to avoid the flood of hormones, the physical disturbance to her body, the pain of childbirth, the dangers to her health, etc., would not, *prima facie,* be acting unethically. And, I agree with Firestone that having the choice could be very liberating for women. But, it would be unlikely to be so in the current social climate.

I do not pretend to predict the future, but the immediate application of this technology in this society's current environment *will* perpetuate the motherhood view of women; the restrictive view rather than the expansive one of encouraging fulfillment of the full range of human potential for all. If advances continue, the option will be extremely attractive to many infertile couples; couples who have developed their responses to infertility in a society which finds infertility a disability, an error, a malady.

This society continues to pressure women to think of themselves as destined to be mothers, encourages men to assume the same, and presumes that the primary caretaking duties will belong to mothers. Exceptions arise, but these stereotypes remain. Such socializing emphasizes women's reproductive value, while devaluing those without this capacity (who must rely on technology in order to become mothers).

Ectogenesis is not likely to be a way to free women from being valued by their society mostly for their wombs. It will not increase the potential for women's non-reproductive contributions to gain in stature. Without a corresponding dissolution of the patriarchal structures of society which would include a deemphasis on the nuclear family and an environment in which the majority of researchers were alert to the ramifications of gender injustice in their research, Firestone would not be hopeful.

5. The Matter of Control

Firestone suggests that two phenomena must occur in order to free women to thrive. Women must be freed from reproductive tyranny by technology *and* the control of that technology must be effectively removed from the present hands. Such removal, Firestone understood, would require the not-insignificant task of restructuring the entire society. Firestone's revolution is perhaps as far away as ever, but I find her view worth pondering. If we are a society committed to equality for all, the challenges embodied in Firestone's work should not be dismissed without analysis. In the last few decades, our society has indeed taken significant strides toward the equality of women. Much, however, remains to be done, and it is my view that ectogenesis will not be immediately helpful.

For Firestone in 1970, and I believe this holds true today as well, "in the hands of our current society and under the direction of current scientists (few of whom are female or even feminist), any attempted use of technology to 'free' anybody is suspect."[11] While the current development of ectogenesis is not meant to "free" anybody, except, certainly, the parents of premature infants from grief, the underlying theme of Firestone's work remains applicable. Any scientific or technological development that takes place within a society which has avoided examining and coming to grips with the failings of its more repressive and oppressive structures will be destined to become tools of those flawed structures.

More specifically, a society which has not reflected on the imperfections implicit in the nuclear family, has not abandoned its undervaluation of things historically labeled "feminine," has remained committed to an unexamined reliance on and lack of compensation for the reproductive labor of women—has, fundamentally, failed to reconstitute itself outside of patriarchal limitations—will not be capable of attaining gender justice through advances in the reproductive industry or any other mechanism.

Any attempts to use technology to free women "from the tyranny of their reproductive biology"[12] requires that control of that technology be in the hands of individuals who will seek to encourage the use of the full range of human potential in women *or* men who choose to reproduce in this way. I can imagine a scientist who would not make stereotypical judgments regarding the range of possibilities of the recipients of his or her research. I can imagine a researcher or clinician who would encourage women *not* to think of themselves as fulfilled only upon completion of a successful pregnancy, who would not be bewildered by a man who wanted nothing more than to take the primary role in raising a child. I can imagine a developer of an artificial womb who would market her or his product as an alternative to the current cumbersome, deforming, excruciating process that it is without tapping into the stereotypes that our society currently embraces with such vigor. I can imagine all of these things, but I do not find them very likely at present.

I do not want to leave the impression that I do not value motherhood. In many of its manifestations it is a richly rewarding and wonderfully efficacious means of raising members of the next generation, and enriching one's own life. Fathers too give themselves the ultimate gift when they play the primary role in their children's lives. My concern, and the thrust of this paper, involves the tunnel vision society uses to gaze on its female members, restricting their growth by encouraging them to define themselves too narrowly. For those kinds of problems, ectogenesis will likely be no help.

NOTES

1. Shulamith Firestone, *The Dialectic of Sex: The Case for Feminist Revolution* (New York: Bantam Books, 1970), p. 206.

2. See for example Mary O'Brien, *The Politics of Reproduction* (Boston: Routledge and Kegan Paul, 1983); Janice Raymond, *Women as Wombs: Reproductive Technologies and the Battle over Women's Freedom* (San Francisco: HarperSanFrancisco, 1983); Gena Corea, *The Mother Machine: Reproductive Technologies from Artificial Insemination to Artificial Wombs* (New York: Harper and Row, 1985).

3. Christine Overall, "Selective Termination of Pregnancy and Women's Reproductive Autonomy," *Hastings Center Report* 20 (May-June 1990), pp. 6–11.

4. See for example J. E. Tyson et al., "Viability, Morbidity, and Resource Use among Newborns of 501-to 800-g Birth Weigh," *JAMA* 276 (1996), pp. 1645–1651; and E. B. St. John et al, "Cost of Neonatal Care according to Gestational Age at Birth and Survival Status," *American Journal of Obstetrics and Gynecology* 182 (2000), pp. 170–175.

5. See R. A. Caldwell, *The Costs of Child Abuse vs. Child Abuse Prevention: Michigan's Experience* (East Lansing, Mich.: Michigan Children's Trust Fund, 1992); M. Massey-Stokes and B. Lanning, "The Role of CSHPs in Preventing Child Abuse and Neglect," *Journal of School Health* 74 (August 2004), p. 2; C. Bruner, *Potential Returns on Investment from a Comprehensive Family Center Approach in High-Risk Neighborhoods: Background Paper, Allegheny County Study* (Des Moines, Iowa: Child and Family Policy Center, 1996); M. S. Gould and T. O'Brien, *Child Maltreatment in Colorado: The Value of Prevention and the Cost of Failure to Prevent* (Denver: Center for Human Investment Policy, University of Colorado at Denver, 1995).

6. Sarah Franklin, "The Dialectic of Sex: Shulamith Firestone Revisited," text published online by the Department of Sociology of Lancaster University, online at http://www.comp.lancs.ac.uk/sociology/papers/word%20docs/franklin-dialectic-of-sex.doc and accessed on 22 August 2001.

7. Elizabeth Bartholet, "In Vitro Fertilization: The Construction of Infertility and Parenting." in *Issues in Reproductive Technology I: An Anthology*, ed. Helen B. Holmes (New York: Garland Publishing, 1992), pp. 253–260.

8. Bartholet, "In Vitro Fertilization: The Construction of Infertility and Parenting," p. 255 (emphasis hers).

9. Franklin, "The Dialectic of Sex: Shulamith Firestone Revisited," p. 2.

10. But see Mary Midgley, "Biotechnology and Monstrosity: Why We Should Pay Attention to the 'Yuk Factor'," *Hastings Center Report* 30 (September-October 2000), pp. 7–15.

11. Firestone, *The Dialectic of Sex*, p. 206.

12. *Ibid.*

Ten

LEAVING PEOPLE ALONE: LIBERALISM, ECTOGENESIS, AND THE LIMITS OF MEDICINE

Dien Ho

In this chapter, I contend that the value arguments against ectogenesis advanced by Leon Kass and Julien Murphy have been largely misunderstood. The inability to justify the moral significance of values by rational arguments poses no threat to their arguments, contrary to Peter Singer's claim. In the face of competing values without a clear winner, however, our actual commitment to respecting individual autonomy as the default position entails that ectogenesis ought not to be prohibited.

1. Introduction

Recent developments in prenatal and neonatal care have established the strong possibility of artificial gestation, or ectogenesis. In its most complete form, ectogenesis allows the entire growth of a fetus to take place outside a woman's womb. How should we evaluate the morality of ectogenesis? What are the central questions that we should address?

I will examine arguments offered by Leon Kass and Julien Murphy that claim that ectogenesis undermines some of our most important values, such as the value of natural birth. I contend that our willingness to integrate new technologies into our lives does not prove our blind faith in science. Nor is it a result of what Kass has so frequently attacked as liberal cowardice (i.e., those who merely "sit in the tub while the water gets hot"). Instead, the expansion of medical intervention occurs because of our shared commitment to liberalism in the face of competing values. We recognize that in the absence of a rational argument one way or another, prohibiting an individual's choice proves to be far more costly from a moral point of view than the potential harm that ectogenesis may cause.

The current ectogenesis debate is a conflict of values in which the value arguments advanced by the anti-ectogenesis side have often been mis-understood and under-appreciated. Once we have explicitly comprehended the nature of their arguments, an acceptable method of resolving value debates will bring us to a consensus, as it has in the resolutions of past value conflicts.

2. Value Arguments against Ectogenesis: The Elephant in the Room

Arguments against ectogenesis fall roughly into two camps. First, there are ordinary objections like safety concerns and the justice of allocating scarce resources to experimental care.[1] Second, there are value arguments resulting from the conflict between ectogenesis and some of our important values such as natural pregnancy. Although these two categories are somewhat related (e.g., safety concerns are value conflicts between the benefits of ectogenesis and the commitment to safeguarding patients), I will focus primarily on the second group.

There is little doubt that ectogenesis threatens the traditional family structure by severing the connection between procreation and gestation. I use the term "traditional family" loosely to denote family arrangements that consist of two genetic parents and the woman is the gestational mother. Divorces, surrogate motherhood, and adoption all pose the same threat. In this respect, the challenges posed by ectogenesis differ only in degree. Ectogenesis, however, seems to stand out: it transforms pregnancy into a purely objectifying experience in that no one in the process will ever have a subjective and private (i.e., cannot be shared) interaction with the fetus. No one, for instance, will ever *feel* the fetus growing in a way that the gestational mother does in the traditional situation. The fetus is out in the open allowing all those interested to witness its growth. To put it bluntly, ectogenesis puts the "creation" back in "procreation." If ordinary pregnancies are natural pregnancies in a descriptive sense, then ectogenesis is as unnatural as it gets.

What is so terrible about abandoning natural procreation? Here we find Leon Kass warning us of the potential danger of the new science of baby making:

> But this movement from natural darkness to artificial light has the most profound implications. What we are considering, really, are not merely new ways of beginning individual human lives but also...new ways of life and new ways of viewing life and the nature of man. Man is defined partly by his origins and his lineage; to be bound up with parents, siblings, ancestors, and descendants is part of what we mean by human. By tampering with and confounding these origins and linkages, we are involved in nothing less than creating a new conception of what it means to be human.[2]

Although the consequences of ectogenesis may not as dire as Kass claims, he is correct to notice that natural reproduction is the source of many of our important social relations and our identity. Moreover, ectogenesis clearly represents a great gestalt switch in which we see pregnancy not as a process to be cherished in and of itself but as a potential obstacle that can be gotten rid of.

Some might argue that using an artificial womb to avoid pregnancy is to miss out on an important occasion in life.

Criticism of ectogenesis comes not only from medical conservatives like Kass. Feminists highlight other serious moral implications. According to Julien Murphy, ectogenesis (or in her terms *in vitro* gestation or IVG) threatens to place greater control on pregnant women:

> First, pregnancy might come to be viewed as an inferior act. Women choosing pregnancy over IVG ... might be seen as taking unnecessary risks with fetal life in order to have an experience of childbirth. Or pregnant women might feel the need to monitor their pregnancies and limit their lives in an attempt to duplicate as much as possible IVG conditions. We might come to see pregnancy as a mere biological function, repeatable in IVG, and not also as a human bond in formation of new life that can be had in no other way.[3]

We should take care to ensure that these consequences are not merely possible (as in what *might* be the case) but likely given ectogenesis. Otherwise, Murphy runs the risk of trivializing her conclusion. Regardless of whether or not one is sympathetic to the implications for our values that she claims, not to take them seriously in determining the morality of ectogenesis is to overlook significant factors. The values are elephants in the room: you might not like the fact that they are there but you cannot simply ignore them.

Suppose ectogenesis does threaten some of our central values. It does not follow deductively that ectogenesis is wrong. In general, if engaging in X will lead to Y and Y eliminates some significant values, it does not follow that X is immoral. Imagine a patient whose legs must be amputated because of gangrene. Although the amputation may leave him unable to walk again (something we ordinarily value a great deal), it does not follow that the amputation is wrong, because not doing so will likely lead to an outcome worse than loss of limbs.

Moreover, if the value argument takes ordinary practices and concludes that they are morally good, then it commits the naturalistic fallacy. The move here leaves one wondering both why this particular set of practices enjoys moral protection and how exactly we go from what is the case to what ought to be the case.

In light of these difficulties, and arguing against the opponents of *in vitro* fertilization, Peter Singer suggests:

> Once the stigma has gone from the fact that IVF does not occur in the normal course of things, to point out that IVF is unnatural in the descriptive sense is to point out nothing which is at all damaging.[4]

Such "brushing off" of the value argument, I think, misses something subtle and powerful about the argument. The proponents of the value argument (including Kass and Murphy) need not justify why they assign values to these practices. Rather, all they have to do is to demonstrate that we in fact assign substantial (not necessary high) value to some practices and that engaging in a certain medical procedures will threaten these values. These two facts constitute a *prima facie* reason to avoid the procedures in question. The beauty of values is that they often do not require justification.

Examples of the non-rational nature of values are abundant in ordinary lives. Consider the difficulty in explaining to someone why Jean-Honoré Fragonard's paintings are deeply moving or why one assigns sentimental value to an old watering hole. Or take the fact that children often reject a replacement toy, even when it is identical to the lost one, because the replacement is "just not the same." When we encounter a foreign culture for the first time and witness their apparently bizarre rituals, we do not ask them to justify the value of their rituals before extending our respect. Instead we immediately respect them because they are important to the practitioners. In this sense, we understand why many readers are sympathetic to Kass's "wisdom of repugnance." In arguing against cloning, Kass writes,

> Yet repugnance need not stand naked before the bar of reason. The wisdom of our horror at human cloning can be partially articulated, even if this is finally one of those instances about which the heart has its reasons that reason cannot entirely know.[5]

I would go further to say that sometimes the heart needs no reason to hold certain values. When doing ethics, we do not operate on a social *tabula rasa*. People have preexisting values that occupy different spaces. To ignore them entirely is to plow through a rich landscape, oblivious to all its rich and subtle features.

3. Ectogenesis as a Conflict of Values

Having said all that, I am not suggesting that values are incorrigible. Nor am I saying that we should maintain them without any critical awareness. Our history testifies that "cultural preservation" often leads to some of the worst injustices. What I am suggesting is that the frustration of the proponents of the value argument can best be explained by the fact that all too often we fail to understand the point of their arguments. They do not aim to show deductively that ectogenesis is immoral on the grounds that it threatens some of our deeply held values; rather, the point is to identify the value conflicts that ectogenesis presents and to ask whether or not ectogenesis is justifiable in light of its potential disruption to our preexisting social fabric. This strategy is plainly overlooked by Peter Singer in his analysis of objections against ectogenesis. Singer identifies four primary objections: (1) ectogenesis may not be safe for the child; (2) ectogenesis undermines some conceptions of womanhood; (3) ectogenesis is unnatural; and (4) ectogenesis represents a slippery step toward a Brave New World-type society.[6] The last three objections, he argues, substantially differ from the first one and he believes that (2)–(4) can easily be dismissed because there are no acceptable readings of "naturalness" that deductively entail the moral impermissibility of ectogenesis. The only genuine question left is whether ectogenesis is safe.

Singer's analysis of the objections against ectogenesis entirely fails to grasp the force of the value argument. Contrary to Singer, I argue that there are in fact no differences in kind between (1) and (2)–(4). They are *all* conflicts of values. After all, why should safety be the only important value that is worth considering? If it is in fact the case that ectogenesis will likely eliminate, say, the value of natural motherhood, why should we entirely leave out this value in our consideration? Our valuing safety is perhaps derived from a more fundamental commitment not to expose patients to unnecessary harm. If this is so, how are we to justify the latter? My suspicion is that it will be no less difficult to justify the value of safety than it is to justify those values that Singer dismisses. Indeed, it appears that the very same set of arguments Singer uses to dismiss the value arguments should also apply to the considerations that he believes are legitimate. By swinging a heavy meta-ethics bat, Singer might have unknowingly demolished his own analysis.

The best way to understand the ectogenesis debate is to see it as a clash between certain fundamental values. On the one hand, we acknowledge the central role natural procreation plays in our web of values; on the other hand, we see that a ban of ectogenesis will clearly jeopardize our commitment to procreative autonomy. Given the fact that no one has a rational argument to convince her opponents that she has the right set of values, the ectogenesis debate, like so many other bioethical debates, remains at an impasse. The worst thing we can do at this junction is to ignore the values put forth by the other side and pound our fists insisting on our own position. In so doing, we gain little ground and convince our opponents that we do not acknowledge values that they believe we hold, thus widening the gulf between the two sides.

4. An Appeal to Liberalism

Although debates of values can easily turn into philosophical "trench warfare" in which no one is expected to make any spectacular gain, we need not be mired in a war of attrition. The reason is that, as a matter of fact, we share some fundamental beliefs as a community about what to do when confronting an apparently irresolvable conflict of values.

Take a relatively uncontroversial example of two groups of individuals who differ in terms of how they believe their children ought to be raised. The first group believes that the ideal childrearing method is to maximize the child's exposure to intellectual activities. The second group sees the importance of letting children participate in determining their own upbringing. Suppose further that no one has a clear argument against the other position (e.g., both positions are internally coherent, etc.). Imagine the two groups have to form a policy legislating childrearing. How are they to decide? It seems obvious that the best thing to do in this case is to let each group do what it intends to do and to let the policy remain as "hands-off" as possible. The reason is that we are committed to the view that when there is a conflict of values without a clear winner, individuals should be free to pursue the courses of action that they see fit. This principle is so ingrained in the foundation of a liberal democracy that one is hard pressed to think of a counter-example. It says in essence that we place a premium on individual liberty and that the default position of any value debate is to avoid restricting an individual's autonomy without just reasons. Let us call this "the principle of default autonomy."

Although I have not had the opportunity to pose this question to all the participants in the ectogenesis debate, I venture to say that every one of them subscribes to this principle. My bold conjecture relies on the obvious undesirability of rejecting the principle. To deny it is to say that in a moral debate, we are permitted to allow someone to restrict our range of action without good reasons. If this permission is granted, what then is the point of rational debate? Indeed, we can easily see how a Rawlsian agent standing behind the veil of ignorance would select the principle of default autonomy. Without knowing in advance one's social position, a rational agent is best not to allow arbitrary restrictions of liberty, mindful of the fact that once the veil is lifted, she may find that it is her liberty that is radically curtailed with no just cause.

The opponents to ectogenesis might argue that in light of the substantial value disagreement, we ought to remain conservative and not permit the practice. It is imperative that we understand exactly the nature of the claim. In a nutshell, they are saying "although we have no rational or non-question begging reasons to convince you why you cannot engage in ectogenesis, nevertheless, we will prohibit you from doing so." This line of argument is potentially dangerous because once it is accepted as legitimate anyone can use it to prohibit anything he or she finds unacceptable. No reasonable participants in the ectogenesis debate could possibly agree to this. Not Kass, not Murphy, and certainly not Singer. In light of our implicit agreement to find a non-draconian solution, as long as the value conflict remains at a standstill, like it or not, ectogenesis should be available.

5. Some Qualifications

It is important to keep in mind that I am not advocating a general normative ethical theory. My point here is simply to show that the gulf between the two sides is smaller than we think. Specifically, our commitment to the principle of default autonomy provides us with the common ground to solve the debate. I do not take this principle to be universally true (although if there are any moral truths, I suspect this is one of them) because I have not supplied an argument to establish it.

My argument is only that we all share the principle as an empirical and contingent matter. The solution that I propose in favor of ectogenesis would not be available if this were not so. In any case, it is safe to say that no arguments are likely to convince someone who does not accept the principle. That means, in essence, she has abandoned the most important ground rule—individuals' freedoms are curtailed only in the face of good reasons.

Likewise, I have taken for granted that we in fact hold many of the values identified by Kass and Murphy and that ectogenesis poses a probable threat to them. If neither claim is correct, then there is no genuine conflict of values, and ectogenesis is drastically less problematic. Indeed, in considering some of the value arguments, one notices the overwhelming number of speculative claims touting the potential dangers of ectogenesis (or whatever new technology is at stake). We are told that if X is available, then it *might* be the case that A and it *might* be the case that B and so on, where A and B are supposedly sacrifices we must make if we engage in X. Speculative premises only deliver speculative conclusions. The problem is that for every speculation that ectogenesis might result in some horrible consequences, we can likewise imagine it strengthening other positive consequences. Recall Murphy's worry that ectogenesis will place further pressure on pregnant women. What about the possibility that it might permit the traditionally non-gestating partner to share the responsibility of fetal development in a more equitable fashion?

Speculations are not sufficient. We need evidence to establish the dangers of ectogenesis and we will not know what they are until it becomes a reality. Is this a problem? No, because we have done this before. We must anticipate ramifications as fully as possible and guide the practice with skill, exactly as we did in making obstetric anesthesia available, or in legalizing *in vitro* fertilization, or in permitting surrogate motherhood. Ectogenesis is merely a point in the history of medical progress. As in the past we have appealed to autonomy, caution, and planning to lead us through the advent of a new technology, we can do likewise with ectogenesis. The fact that we are still here with all of our human splendors and defects should positively testify to our method of resolving value conflicts.

6. Lost in Space or the Best of All Possible Worlds?

Opponents to medical progress, especially to procreative technologies, have often expressed a sense of helplessness in the face of science. They feel that somehow we are too eager to embrace the promise of a better medicine while not taking into consideration its impact on our nature. I think there is a misunderstanding here. Kass begins the chapter titled "Making Babies" in his book *Towards a More Natural Science* with the following quotation:

> Good afternoon ladies and gentleman. This is your pilot speaking. We are flying at an altitude of 35,000 feet and a speed of 700 miles an hour. I have two pieces of news to report, one good and one bad. The bad news is that we are lost. The good news is that we are making very good time.[7]

Rather than seeing ourselves as heading nowhere fast, I would instead think of the direction of medicine as one explicitly guided by the principle of rational resolution in the face of conflicting values. The reality is that we know exactly where we are heading at each junction because we deliberate and anticipate the course ahead. What Kass is really pointing out is that we often do not like our destinations but he fails to understand that the alternatives are far worse. We remain moral beings because we stand by our philosophical principles. If we are to make policy decisions driven by ethical considerations, then we should be prepared for consequences that we might not like. After all, what is the point of ethics if we always like what is right?

7. Conclusion

Those who advance value arguments against ectogenesis are justified in feeling misunderstood. Their positions have been dismissed too quickly on the ground they cannot rationally support why they assign values to the social practices in question. The fact of the matter is that they need not do that. All they have to establish is that these values are important to us and as such they have to be given *prima facie* moral force. Moreover, when those like Singer dismiss the anti-ectogenesis value arguments in favor of liberal values, the opponents of ectogenesis rightly notice the hypocrisy involved and demand to know why exclusively liberal values are considered.

This chapter's analysis places the value arguments in the proper perspective by recognizing the moral importance of values advocated by the anti-ectogenesis side. In order to move past the stalemate, we appeal to a deeper commitment to the principle of letting individuals choose for themselves when no just reasons are given to limit their autonomy. My belief is that all sides subscribe to the principle of default autonomy and that ectogenesis ought to be permitted based on this tried and true methodology. I have intentionally left out other important issues in my analysis such as the impact of ectogenesis on the abortion debate. My aim, however, is only to reconcile some of the value arguments (specifically, the conflict between ectogenesis and our conceptions of ourselves) and I leave untouched how ectogenesis will mesh with other ethical views.

NOTES

1. See David N. James, "Ectogenesis: A Reply to Singer and Wells," *Bioethics* 1 (1987): 80–99.
2. Leon R. Kass, *Toward a More Natural Science* (New York: Free Press, 1985), p. 48.
3. Julien S. Murphy, "Is Pregnancy Necessary? Feminist Concerns About Ectogenesis," *Hypatia* 4 (1989), p. 79 [this volume, pp. 39–40].
4. Peter Singer and Deane Wells, *Making Babies: The New Science and Ethics of Conception* (New York: Charles Scribner's Sons, 1985), p. 38.
5. Leon R. Kass and James Q. Wilson, *The Ethics of Human Cloning* (Washington, D.C.: AEI Press, 1998), p. 24.
6. Singer and Wells, *Making Babies*, pp. 124–126 [this volume, pp. 16–18].
7. Kass, *Toward a More Natural Science*, p. 43.

Eleven

IMMACULATE GESTATION? HOW WILL ECTOGENESIS CHANGE CURRENT PARADIGMS OF SOCIAL RELATIONSHIPS AND VALUES?

Jennifer S. Bard

1. Introduction

Given the pace of medical research in the last ten years, there is no technology that seems out of reach no matter how ethically questionable or absurd. Many interventions and procedures we now take for granted, such as blood transfusions, heart transplants, ultrasound imaging and fetal surgery, are examples of science fiction becoming reality. This explosion of new technology foretells the likelihood of a serious challenge to the law of abortion if human reproduction no longer requires the active participation by two persons of the opposite sex. One such technology, so far not perfected, is the gestation of a human being outside of the womb. Ectogenesis calls into question what has been the immutable fact of reproduction from the beginning of time: A fetus must gestate in a woman's body. The best place to look for a legal analogy to ectogenesis are in cases considering frozen embryos and posthumous sperm donation, two technologies that already alter the natural process of reproduction. Previewing the issue of a woman's right to voluntarily terminate a pregnancy, both frozen embryo and posthumous sperm donation cases consider a person's right not to reproduce even though some steps towards conception have already occurred.

What is interesting about these technological advances is that the law of abortion as fashioned by the Supreme Court is rooted in what has been until now the immutable biological facts of human reproduction. As we see these facts changing we will need to re-evaluate the interpretation of the constitution that finds a woman's right to abortion as the right to control her body.

One of the much-discussed futuristic technologies is the development of an ectogenesis mechanism, reminiscent of that in Huxley's *Brave New World*,[1] to gestate a human fetus outside the human body in an artificial womb. The impact of ectogenesis on social relationships and values would be greater than the extraordinary reproductive technologies developed within the last twenty years. This article will discuss how the law's view of the mother's and father's legal rights would be affected by the existence of technology that would gestate a fetus outside of the body from conception to birth.

2. Factual Background

A normal pregnancy is 40 weeks. Babies born before 37 weeks are called preterm. The current state of medical technology has advanced so as to sustain a baby born as early as 23 or 24 weeks after gestation. Before the 23 or 24 week period, the ability to sustain a baby outside the womb quickly drops to zero. Ectogenesis is, then, the logical end of a continuum that has been developing into full panoply of incubators and equipment already in use to support premature infants. For example, extra corporeal membrane oxygenation, which bypasses the heart and oxygenates blood outside of the body, has become routine.[2]

Seen as an improvement of current efforts to save premature babies, the benefits of a safe and effective form of ectogenesis would be extensive. No one imagines that the current incubators are any more than a crude attempt to reproduce womb conditions so that preterm infants can grow strong enough to survive in the outside world. Beyond improving the chances of survival of the babies now eligible for incubator support, an artificial womb offers opportunities to save embryos at any stage who cannot survive in the womb environment they are born into.

For the purposes of discussion, this paper will consider ectogenesis in its pure form, which would be the ability to gestate a zygote from conception to birth outside the womb. Ectogenesis will probably develop progressively, working back from the current high technology that allows keeping babies alive who have only spent 23 or 24 weeks in the womb.

3. Analysis

The invention of a method to gestate a baby outside the human womb has enormous implications for the way the courts, ethicists and society at large currently view the right of a fetus to be born. It also influences how society thinks about the relationship between the fetus and its parents. One issue that exemplifies the strain on social relationships is the right of a mother or father to end the life of a fetus at some point prior to birth. In the case of *in vitro* fertilization there is one moment in time, when the fetus can be given a chance at life, implanted, or discarded. At this point, the fetus is an independent living being, separate from the body of both mother and father. Ectogenesis stretches out this moment into a nine-month continuum. Because the fetus is gestated outside of the womb there is no longer any reason to priviledge a mother's right to terminate a pregnancy over the father's since both mothers and fathers have made biologically equivalent contributions towards the creation of a new life.

A. Would the Availability of Ectogenesis Give Every Fetus a Right to Life?

The law of abortion is a delicate balancing act based on an unstable premise that the mother's rights to control over her body trump the rights of a fetus to be born alive up until a certain mysterious point where the rights of the embryo take on independent significance. Over the last thirty years the Supreme Court of the United States has grappled with the issue of balancing the right of the state in potential life versus the right of a woman to have control over her body. The leading Supreme Court cases interpreting the legal standards for abortion are *Roe v. Wade*, 410 U.S. 113, 93 S.Ct.705, 35 L.Ed.2d 147(1973), *Planned Parenthood of Southeastern Pennsylvania v. Casey*, 505 U.S. 833, 112 S.Ct. 2791, 120 L.Ed.2d 674 (1992); and *Stenberg v. Carhart*, 530 U.S. 914, 120 S.Ct. 2597, 147 L.Ed.2d 743 (2000). Each subsequent decision was influenced by the then current state of medical technology.

The current paradigm for judging a fetus's right to life is that rights increase as viability becomes more likely. For instance, a Washington, D.C. court weighed viability in considering a petition to order that a cesarean delivery be performed on a dying woman carrying a fetus which was theoretically old enough to survive outside the womb.[3] In concluding that the cesarean should be performed in the face of what had been earlier refusals of the surgery by the mother, the court wrote, "The child's interest in being born with as little impairment as possible should also be considered.... The most important factor on this side of the scale, however, is life itself, because the viable unborn child that dies because of the mother's refusal to have a caesarean delivery is deprived, entirely and irrevocably, of the line on which the child was about to embark."

If technology advances to a point that every fetus was viable at every stage of development how can society permit abortion? To some extent this has happened with the *Casey* Court's abandonment of the *Roe v. Wade* trimester test in favor of a viability standard. Stressing viability, the *Stenberg* Court acknowledged that a woman had a constitutional right to an abortion; but that the State has an equal right to regulate abortion even if the intent is to discourage it.

Although the trimester standard has been abandoned, there is still at the core of abortion law a belief that there is some point during gestation which marks the time before which a fetus can be aborted. This principle is based on the fundamental unfairness of forcing a woman to gestate a child. However, if gestation were not an issue, abortion law might look very different. If ectogenesis was fully developed, it could replace the current necessity of a fetus to gestate in a womb. In cases like the one in Washington where the fetus needs to be removed from a womb, ectogenesis would allow the pregnancy to continue in a nurturing environment.

A further implication of ectogenesis is that any fertilized egg could be gestated outside of the human body at any time in the fetus's development. Thus, a four-day-old fertilized zygote could be gestated to term without the aid of a woman willing to undergo implantation and then pregnancy. Just as interesting, a mother who chose not to continue a pregnancy at any stage could have the fetus transferred to an artificial womb where development would proceed to birth. Can the concept of viability survive in a world where every fertilized egg can be gestated without the direct involvement of a human being?

It seems a short leap from the ability to continue a pregnancy in an artificial womb to the requirement that every unwanted pregnancy must be completed in an artificial womb. From a utilitarian point of view, the value of an increase in the number of infants born is highly variable. In the United States this might mean more infants available for adoption. Currently in the United States demand for adoptable babies far exceeds supply, but there is no reason to think that demand is very large. In considering the issue of forced gestation we must be very conscious of the culture and class which inform our beliefs. In India or China the proposition that every embryo deserves life would result in a disastrous population explosion that would soon exhaust already limited resources. Even in the United States some babies are more adoptable than others.

At the heart of the abortion issue is the question: what is a person? Some of the most important thinking and writing on the issue of whether an embryo has the same rights as a post-birth human have been done by Judith Jarvis Thomson[4] and Peter Singer.[5] In "A Defense of Abortion" Thomson develops the premise that an adult will die unless he is "connected" to the body of a healthy woman for nine months. This connection, called "plugging in" by Thomson, is described as somewhat risky, but mostly inconvenient and uncomfortable. Why, asks Thomson, should the needs of one person, no matter how great, require another person to serve as his life support system? In Thomson's example the man has already been born. Being in that state, does he have a right to remain alive? Not, she concludes if it means making use of another's body. She writes "having a right to life does not guarantee having either a right to be given the use of or a right to be allowed continued use of another person's body—even if one needs it for life itself."

Peter Singer offers a utilitarian criticism of Thomson's hypothetical. He states that if the consequences of disconnection are "worse than the consequences of remaining connected" the host, willing or unwilling, should remain connected. He argues that if a fetus, like an adult, has a protected interest and that right must be exercised through use of another's body then it "would be wrong to refuse to carry the fetus until it can survive outside the womb."[6] He argues that the host body could refuse to serve as a life-support system, but that such refusal would be wrong.

In rejecting Thomson's arguments on utilitarian grounds, Singer also rejects the concept of a fetus' right to life. He argues that anyone willing to kill an animal for meat cannot protest the killing of an unborn child because both are of equal value. He also writes that a fetus has no more rights than an animal because it is unconscious and not rational.

A corollary to Singer's thesis is that if animals were afforded a right to life, then the fetus should be as well. It is not necessary to agree with Singer's criteria for personhood to conclude that personhood is an extremely complex concept about which many thoughtful people disagree.

B. Without Pregnancy, Would a Mother's Rights To Make Decisions About Her Unborn Child Still Prevail Over a Father's Rights?

Without deciding the definition of personhood, the Supreme Court held in its consideration of abortion in 2000 (*Stenberg v. Carhart*) that a woman's right was "to decide to terminate a pregnancy free of undue interference by State." At the same time, the court recognized that the state has a right to enact laws favoring life.

Traditionally, the difference between a woman's rights and a man's rights rest on the biological fact that it is the woman who must gestate and give birth to the baby. With pregnancy removed from the equation, men and women stand on equal ground. This has begun to be recognized in cases where mothers and fathers disagree on the disposition of their frozen embryos.

Recent cases about frozen embryo ownership support the idea that a mother or a father may choose for their embryo not to be born. In *Davis v. Davis*, 84 S.W. 2d 588 (1992) the Supreme Court of Tennessee wrote that the man and woman who were the genetic parents of six frozen embryos "must be seen as entirely equivalent gamete providers." The court concluded "none of the concerns about a woman's bodily integrity that have previously precluded men from controlling abortion decisions is applicable here." While the court recognized that the process of IVF (*in vitro* fertilization) was more invasive and stressful for the woman "their experience ... must be viewed in light of the joys of parenthood that is desired or the relative anguish of a lifetime of unwanted parenthood."

In a recent decision involving custody of frozen embryos the New Jersey Supreme Court recognized both the mother's and the father's claim.[7] The mother was allowed to prevent the implantation of the embryos against the father's objections. The justification for this decision was not that such prevention was a mother's prerogative, but rather that no one, neither a mother nor father, should be forced to procreate. The rights of fathers, as viewed by the

Supreme Court, are well summarized by Mary Lyndon Shelley in her book *Making Babies, Making Families.*[8]

C. Posthumous Sperm Donation

The issue of control over reproduction arises again in the growing body of law surrounding posthumous births. It has long been technically possible to store frozen sperm. Increasingly, this is being done by men before undergoing cancer therapy which might make them infertile. The latest advancement is the practice of actually extracting sperm from a man who has died recently and then freezing the sperm for future use.

But who is entitled to use the sperm? Courts in the United States and Europe have grappled with the question of the dead father's control over future use of his sperm. A California court ruled that a man who had committed suicide had expressed his intent for his girlfriend to bear his child posthumously.[9] The girlfriend was awarded custody of the sperm. Similarly the New Jersey Supreme Court upheld a wife's right to bear her husband's children posthumously based on his previous consent.[10] While the decisions in the United States have approved of posthumous conception because of the father's explicit consent, in Europe where such consent has been absent conception has not been allowed.

In England, a court refused to allow a widow access to her dead husband's sperm because he died before giving permission for posthumous conception. Although the court recognized that the man and his wife had been "actively trying to start a family" the man died without banking sperm or leaving instructions.[11] In another case in England, a wife was denied use of her husband's banked sperm because he had withdrawn his written consent for posthumous conception.[12]

Even if the mother and father agree on an abortion, the existence of ectogenesis may give the state grounds to override their decision. For example, one view of the right to abortion is that it is legally and ethically permissible not to bring a severely handicapped infant into the world. The "rights" of women to make the decision to abort a handicapped baby are rolled into her general right to have an abortion for any reason. But what if the infant was not in her body? Would parents still be able to make the value decision that some babies with genetic handicaps should be denied gestation? Could the state be allowed to make decisions on what lives are worth living? Could an individual doctor? Would an ethics committee become involved? Would we not be back exactly where we were when committees decided who got dialysis based on social as much as medical criteria?

Where would the selection stop? At Downs syndrome, at deafness, at shortness? And what if the parents disagreed with the committee's decision?

The situation is equally difficult from the converse perspective. What if the state set some minimum standards of health for a fetus to be allowed access to ectogenesis? Could parents insist, as they can now, that the most hopelessly impaired child be gestated to birth on the grounds that every life is precious? Who would pay for the care? Could a private insurer refuse to cover the medical costs of a handicapped child? How different is that from the current situation in which some health insurance companies will not pay for genetic screening unless the parents are willing to consider terminating the pregnancy? Would the funding source—whether it be public or private at that time—be able to make the decision? In *Stenberg v. Carhart* the Supreme Court held that a woman's right was "to decide to terminate a pregnancy free of undue interference by State." At the same time the Court recognized that the state has a right to enact laws favoring life. The key question is: Could the state enact laws terminating a life by overriding a decision made by the parents and doctors?

Having mentioned severe handicaps it may seem trivial to consider sex selection, but the recent position of the American Society of Reproductive Medicine that sex selection is an appropriate reason to discard a pre-implantation embryo brings the issue to the table.[13]

The acting chairman of the ASRM "used the term 'gender variety' to explain the acceptable uses of sex selection techniques." A parent who already had a boy (or two boys) could select only to have female embryos implanted. It also leads to the question of why gender variety is an acceptable reason for sex selection in the United States but sex selection for males only is viewed as an immoral practice when exercised in China or India. While the repercussions of this decision are only just beginning to be heard, it is clear that the ASRM was reflecting the views of at least some of its members. Dr. Nobert Gleicher, a fertility specialist whose group has nine centers, reported "we will offer it immediately.... Frankly, we have a list of patients who asked for it." This represents the values of the market place triumphing over the values of individuals.

What ectogenesis does in its purest form is to ask us to re-evaluate all our current legal and ethical theory on the status of a fetus in embryo. Is the embryo property? Is it a person? As courts have struggled with the issue of abortion, no one has been satisfied with the attempts to draw distinctions between the mother's rights and the child's as well.

4. Conclusion: What Will the Future Bring?

Much of the future development of policy depends on how or if ectogenesis would be regulated. Due to the ban on Federal Research on embryos, fertility medicine has fallen almost entirely into the hands of the for profit private sector. The question isn't "should we do this" but rather "will someone pay for this?" As the demand for fertility treatment seems insatiable in the United States, research in the field is funded by a cadre of infertile men and women desperate for children at any price. Here again, the values of the market place may be at odds with the values of society as a whole.

Where does this leave ectogenesis? Is it the promise of a giant leap in medical technology that would save premature infants who are currently either beyond help or severely at risk? Does it require a complete rethinking of a woman's right to choose? Was that right only a fluke of nature? Does the right to choose whether a baby is born vanish when the woman no longer harbors the baby inside of her body?

Ectogenesis will bring about radical change in the way society views social relationships. Fathers will need to be considered on terms equal with mothers since both parents have done no more than permit the fertilization of an egg. What will the state's role be? Will ectogenesis become the latest high cost technology available on the private market for any purpose someone can pay for?

Is it unduly pessimistic to focus the discussion of ectogenesis on un-wanted babies? The increasingly sophisticated techniques and equipment which are the precursors to ectogenesis are all intended to save much wanted children who otherwise could not survive because of their prematurity. Could a technology that can gestate a baby outside the womb be restricted to such high social utility uses as saving micro preemies from a lifetime of expensive care by forestalling the lifelong sequela of prematurity?

On the other hand, would there be any way to stop baby factories in the private sector or, more likely, in resource-scarce third world countries that would provide the use of this technology to anyone who can afford the price?

These issues cannot begin to be resolved until they are discussed completely. There are models for developing a public consensus. For example the previously constituted Presidential Bioethics Advisory Committee sought the public's opinion through open meetings and invitations for comment. In her book *Where Science Offers Salvation*,[14] Rebecca Dresser argues that input from the public is important because they are stakeholders in the result of medical research. She calls for the involvement of health care advocates to represent the public in analyzing research proposals. The need for public involvement in ectogenesis is strengthened by the fact that much of the research involving fetuses in this country is unregulated. Because the Federal Government will not fund embryo research at this time, technological advances are in the hands of for-profit fertility clinics, which combine research and treatment.

There are international models as well for public involvement. In Canada the committee charged with developing cloning polled and interviewed a substantial portion of the population before establishing guidelines.[15] Such public discussion should take place in the United States well in advance of the final perfection of the technology of ectogenesis. That full implementation of ectogenesis does not seem imminent is not reason to ignore its wide-reaching implications.

NOTES

1. Aldous Huxley, *Brave New World and Brave New World Revisited* (New York: Harper and Row, 1965).

2. Jeffrey Pomerance and C. Joan Richardson, *Neonatology for the Clinician* (Norwalk, Conn.: Appleton and Lange, 1993), pp. 325.

3. *In re* A.C., 573 A.2d 1235 (1990).

4. Judith Jarvis Thomson, "A Defense of Abortion" in *Today's Moral Issues*, 2nd ed., ed. Daniel Bonevac (Mountain View, Cal.: Mayfield, 1996), p. 317.

5. Peter Singer, "Taking Life: The Embryo and the Fetus," in *Writings on an Ethical Life* (New York: Harper Collins, 2000), pp. 146–164.

6. Ibid., p. 154.

7. *J.B. v. M.B.*, 2001 NJ.Lexis 955.

8. Mary Lyndon Shanley, *Making Babies, Making Families: What Matters Most in an Age of Reproductive Technologies, Surrogacy, Adoption, and Same-sex and Unwed Parents* (Boston: Beacon Press, 2001), pp. 145–175.

9. *Hecht v. Superior Court*, 16 Cal. App. 4th 836, 20 Cal. Rptr. 2d. 275, 62 USLW 2007 (Cal. App. 2 Dist. Jun 17, 1993) (NO. B073747), review denied (Sep 02, 1993). See also *Woodward v. Comm'r of Social Security*, 435 Mass. 536, 760 N.E. 2d. 257 (2002).

10. *In re Kolacy*, 332 N.J. Super. 593, 753 A.2d 1257 (2001).

11. Embryology Authority, R V. Human Fertilization and Ex Parte Blood, Queen's Bench Division (1996) 3 WLR 1176, 35 BMLR 1 (1997) 2 FLR. 170.

12. *Center for Reproductive Media v. U Court of Appeal* (Civil Division) (2002) EWCA Civ S65. See also *Parpalaix v. Cecos*, T.G.I. Creteil, 1 August 1984, Gaz. du PaL 1984, 2, pan. jurisp., 560.

13. Gina Kolata, "Fertility Authority Approves Sex Selection," *New York Times* (28 September 2001), p. A16.

14. Rebecca Dresser, *When Science Offers Salvation* (New York: Oxford University Press, 2001), pp. 99–108.

15. *Proceed with Care: Final Report of the Royal Commission on New Reproductive Technologies* (Ottawa, Canada: Royal Commission on New Reproductive Technologies, 1993).

Twelve

THE ARTIFICIAL WOMB AND HUMAN SUBJECT RESEARCH

Joyce M. Raskin and Nadav A. Mazor

The artificial womb (AW) has been in the human imagination for more than eighty years. The biologist J. B. S. Haldane is credited with coining the term ectogenesis—out of body birth—in 1924 and in 1932, Aldous Huxley described human gestating machines in his book *Brave New World*. It is only today that current research provides the promise that the technology may be available in the near future. Already, two groups of researchers are attempting to create artificial wombs for the ultimate purpose of reproductive treatment. One group in Japan has successfully managed to transfer fetal goats to an artificial womb made of plastic. This model of artificial womb is intended for complete external gestation. Another group, at Cornell University, has successfully implanted a human in vitro fertilized (IVF) embryo into a womb constructed of endometrial cells taken from the uterine wall of a human female. This model is intended for partial gestation in which the embryo grows externally until the artificial womb and the fetus in it can be wholly transplanted into the woman's body. Further development of the technology may require extensive use of human embryos and fetuses.

As AW research progresses and more human embryos and fetuses are used, it is inescapable that the ethical field of human subject research will have to respond to the challenge presented by the technology. This field of ethics which evaluates research performed on human subjects developed at a time when the definition of a "human subject" seemed more simple and clear: a living human. The artificial womb will impact dramatically on that simple definition. It will force us to reassess what a "human subject" is.

Externally gestated fetuses, implanted in a machine for reproductive purposes, will unavoidably raise the prospect of a new class of human entities that currently do not exist, namely in vitro fetuses. We will need to formulate appropriate standards and guidelines as to what the parameters should be for ethically acceptable research with these new "subjects." Current guidelines regarding research with living humans and research with IVF embryos may offer some insight. However, there are certain aspects to research involving AW that are totally unique and new.

When gestation occurs outside the female body, who, or what, will be considered the subject of the research procedure? Is it the mother, the externally developing fetus, or both? To what extent should informed consent given by parents justify research on an in vitro fetus? What would be the moral status of the in vitro fetus? Should that moral status be different from that which we currently attribute to in vivo fetuses? Should AW research per se, where there is no intention to complete gestation, be allowed?

This chapter poses the question of whether the field of human subject research is sufficiently equipped for, or adaptable to, the challenge of research involving externally existing embryos and/or fetuses. We will review the current bioethical standards governing human subject research on living humans, human embryos, and traditionally gestated human fetuses. Then we will analyze the applicability of the existing guidelines to the development of the artificial womb. Finally, we will suggest necessary adaptations of those guidelines in order to effectively balance between valuable scientific research and the meaning society wishes to attribute to in vitro fetuses.

1. Current Biomedical Standards for Human Subject Research

A. Human Subject Research with Living Humans

Catalytic events inspired the creation of guidelines and protection in the field of human subject research involving living humans. Notably, the inhumane experiments performed on humans by Nazi physicians that led to the Nuremburg tribunal in 1947 served as a strong impetus to question the appropriateness and acceptability of research involving living human subjects. *The Nuremburg Code*,[1] created in response to horrible experimentation practices, laid down ten conditions that must be met before research using human subjects is permissible. The single most important feature of the Code is its first condition, that the *voluntary consent* of the human subject is absolutely essential. It is important to remember that this Code stands for the proposition that research using human subjects is valuable and valid. The fact that these standards were adopted worldwide is an acceptance of that proposition.

Starting from this point, the need for additional guidelines became increasingly evident. A large number of countries, and many international organizations, have promulgated regulations and guidelines for human subject research. For example, the World Medical Association *Declaration of Helsinki*, adopted originally in 1964,[2] deals primarily with physicians conducting human subject research. Based on the nature of the physician's responsibility, as a physician, the Declaration of Helsinki limits the purposes for which biomedical research can be done "to improve prophylactic, diagnostic and therapeutic procedures and the understanding of the aetiology and pathogenesis of disease."[3] The startling discovery in the early 1970s of the Tuskegee syphilis study increased sensitivity to this issue because syphilis researchers used disadvantaged, rural African American males and withheld treatment, even when it was available. This incident, along with others, led to the 1974 National Research Act in the United States which established a commission to identify basic principles relevant to the ethics of human subject research. The commission's *Belmont Report*, published in the United States in 1979, laid down three basic principles relevant to the ethics of research involving human subjects: respect for persons, beneficence, and justice. The idea of respect was that individuals should be treated as autonomous agents capable of judgment and self determination. Informed consent is a natural outgrowth of this. Beneficence is a version of the Hippocratic maxim "Do no harm." One should not seriously harm another person regardless of the benefit that might come to others. Justice is the fairness of distribution of the benefits and risks of medical research.

Over the years the above principles were discussed and applied to various medical research instances where potential harm to living humans was recognizably possible. During that same period of time the focus of the inquiry regarding human subject research shifted from what research was allowable to the question of what and who is being protected. Vulnerable and dependent subjects who needed greater protection were identified. These included prisoners, racial minorities, the critically ill, children and infants. The need to adjust the principles to those specific groups became more and more apparent.

One of the biggest challenges in applying the principles to vulnerable individuals came from an unexpected frontier. The successful application of IVF technology to humans in 1978 created the possibility to achieve a human embryo living outside the human body. The term "human" lost its solid ground. The question of what exactly these entities were became crucial to decide if the principles extended to the new population. Once it was decided that embryos are, to some degree, part of the "human community" the subsequent question was how to adapt the principles to fit their unique status.

B. Human Subject Research and Embryo Research

IVF allowed, for the first time, the observation of human embryo development outside the womb. Enormous medical interest in embryological development raised the concern that not only unused embryos left over from IVF treatments would be used for research but also that embryos might be intentionally created solely for research purposes.

The Warnock Report,[4] published in the United Kingdom in 1984, came about as a direct result of the birth of the first IVF infant. The Committee of Inquiry into Human Fertilisation and Embryology spent two years studying the social, ethical, and legal implications of issues raised by new and potential assisted reproduction technologies for the purpose of making recommendations for legislation. This committee was a fundamental step in attempting to decide how to deal with research involving human embryos. Pertinent findings and recommendations of that Committee, as reported by Mary Warnock include:

- The human embryo *per se* has no legal status. It is not accorded the same status as a living child or adult; nor does it have a right to life. However, the human embryo ought to have a special status and human embryos should be afforded some protection in the law.
- No embryonic research should be made if the purposes of the research could be achieved by the use of other animals or in some other way.
- Research may be carried out on IVF spare embryos only with the informed consent of the parents.
- Intentional creation of embryos for research was a big concern; however, the majority accepted it.
- There should be a limit on the length of time that an embryo can be kept alive in vitro.[5]

After considering a variety of points along the embryonic developmental process that could serve as the time after which an embryo should not be kept alive, the committee recommended that "no live human embryo derived from in vitro fertilization ... may be kept alive, if not transferred to a woman, beyond fourteen days after fertilization, nor may it be used as a research subject beyond fourteen days after fertilization."[6]

Similar committees and studies were established in many countries to address the unique situation that IVF and the new ability to produce embryos for research presented. Many reached the same conclusion as the Warnock Committee, that externally existing embryos were not humans as previously understood in the field of regulation of human subject research. However, the "potential" of such embryos to become humans required a measure of dignity be given them that would be apposite to that afforded humans. In many jurisdictions where this issue was addressed, the choice was made to allow research on human embryos for the first fourteen days only and thereafter ban any research.

The isolation of embryonic stem cells in 1998 made the debate more acute, as the price for extracting the precious master cells was the "potential" life of the embryo. The great promise of the new medical potential to use stem cells to treat and cure diseases such as diabetes, Parkinson's, and Alzheimer's drew the public into the discussion of what the ethical borders for this research should be, perhaps more than any earlier instances of problematic research involving human subjects.

The fourteen day limit on embryonic research is odd from the aspect of human subject research. Embryos used for research are not intended for reproductive purposes and thus will not be implanted and will never become human persons. At approximately fourteen days the blastocyst develops the "primitive streak" and the differentiation stage begins. If at that point the embryo is not implanted it will naturally expire. Karen Dawson explains that at some point the in vitro embryo is different from the in vivo embryo,

> The development of the in vitro pre-embryo up until about seven days after fertilization is roughly equivalent to that in vivo. Beyond this, however, there is no equivalence in development. Development in vitro after this time is more equatable with disorganized cancerous growth. Given this, is a limit on the time over which embryo research can be carried out relevant now? No primitive streak will be formed in in vitro pre-embryos at this stage; so is this entity really deserving of moral status at present? Can it properly be considered to be a pre-embryo?[7]

Why afford total protection to an entity that cannot exist at that point in any case? Does it make sense to totally prohibit research on those embryos, a privilege that fetuses, infants and adults do not have?

Ironically, the fourteen day rule not only fails to protect the naturally dying embryo but actually insures that the embryo will not survive. Would this "protection" make sense if an artificial womb were available for implantation? Complex as the embryo debate may be, the artificial womb presents us with the same hard moral questions but brings them to a new level of discussion as the theater of gestation becomes seeable and its players accessible.

C. Human Subject Research and Fetal Research

The medical definition of a fetus relates to the period of development from eight weeks to birth, eight weeks being generally the point at which the organs and systems have been formed. Research with fetuses in utero has a much longer history than research with IVF embryos (note that abortion was never considered research that falls within the human subject research concepts). Fetal research became an important field in the 1960s, in part because of devastating deformities caused by Thalidomide. It became clear that many substances cross the placental barrier and that animal studies alone were not sufficient to prove a particular drug was safe for the fetus. Thus, fetal research was necessary to test the effect of drugs on fetuses. This research inspired scientists to develop a test for the Rh factor, amniocentesis, and certain types of genetic screening. In the early 1970s researchers also started testing new systems for fetal life support, artificial placentas, and used living but nonviable fetuses for research.

The Supreme Court decision in *Roe v. Wade*[8] provided a constitutional right for a woman to determine whether or not to terminate a pregnancy. This decision gave rise to the concern that abortions would be performed solely for the purpose of fetal research. As a result, the National Research Act was passed in 1974 which banned non-therapeutic fetal research, meaning that research not intended to benefit the fetus, would receive no federal support. The ban was not lifted until 1985 with the Health Research Extension Act. This act was subsequently subsumed by the Code of Federal Regulations (CFR), which governs all federally funded human subject research.[9]

The salient feature of the CFR regarding fetal research is that the provisions regarding research apply throughout the entire gestation period, from conception to birth, a static standard that does not change or increase with development of the fetus. Under this regulation the human fetus, from the time of implantation, enjoys a relatively higher moral status than the IVF embryo and is afforded stronger protection against harmful research. The regulations state explicitly that risks to which a fetus may be subjected are limited to those caused solely by "interventions or procedures that hold out the prospect of direct benefit [therapeutic] for the woman or the fetus; or, if there is no such prospect of benefit [non-therapeutic], the risk to the fetus is not greater than minimal and the purpose of the research is the development of important biomedical knowledge which cannot be obtained by any other means."[10]

Since the CFR defines "fetus" as "the product of conception from *implantation* to delivery"[11] we find that at the early stage of development, human embryos obtain different moral protection depending on whether they are implanted in a womb or not. We learn that the mere existence of an embryo in a womb adds value to its moral status. The same embryo in a Petri dish has less ethical standing and may be exposed to intrusive experiments, even destructive ones. The question thus arises, why does the *implantation* in a womb increase the moral status and therefore afford better protection? What is it about the womb that makes the difference?

Notably, in vivo fetuses are generally not exposed to harmful research due to the fact that they dwell in a pregnant woman's womb, inaccessible to scientists and researchers without her consent. Obviously the mother is the best protector against intrusive and risky research on the fetus. But more than that, it seems that due to the fact that the in vivo fetus is gestated in a living human's body, it benefits from this human's full moral status. For research purposes, it is hard to distinguish between the two entities because the pregnant mother and the fetus are physically inseparable. It is doubtful that the current guidelines treat the fetus on its own.

Clearly the CFR and similar ethical standards applicable to fetuses relate only to a fetus growing in a natural uterus. They do not anticipate fetal development occurring outside the womb. How would human subject research regulations and guidelines gauge the moral status of a fetus that grows in an artificial womb machine, physically separated from a female body? Would such a fetus receive different protection than the in vivo one? How much moral weight should we assign to the mere act of implantation, once it also can be done artificially?

2. Human Subject Research and In Vitro Fetuses

An in vitro fetus does not fall within the definition of any of the unborn entities we know today. It is different from the current IVF embryo, although both develop externally from a living human body. The major difference between the IVF embryo and the in vitro fetus is one of expected development. IVF is a reproductive technology limited to fertilization, or conception, not gestation. If not implanted, the IVF embryo will naturally die less than fourteen days. On the other hand, the in vitro fetus growing in an AW has already initiated the process of gestation, thereby will continue to develop and reach full term within an external environment. Thus its development is not limited in time. Also, unlike the IVF embryo in a petri dish, which is a mass of undifferentiated cells resembling a mulberry, the in vitro fetus develops body organs and is on its way to becoming much more recognizable as a human being.

Although similar in development to the in vivo fetus, the in vitro fetus is also different from that entity. First, and foremost, the in vitro fetus is not embedded within a human body relying on nourishment from body in order to develop. In that sense, the in vitro fetus can be considered more independent than the in vivo fetus. This independent nature of gestation leads to a second, potentially legal and moral difference, viability. Currently the U.S. Supreme court and several state legislatures use the concept of viability to impute legal and moral status for a developing fetus. Language such as "the ability to exist outside the womb albeit with artificial aid" or "meaningful life outside the mother's womb" is used to describe viability as a point of development at which the fetus comes within the ambit of state interest.[12] Thus, because it exists outside the womb with artificial aid, the in vitro fetus could *technically* be considered viable, and therefore receive higher protection, much earlier than the in vivo fetus.

An additional aspect to the consideration of viability is our understanding of the moment at which birth occurs. The traditional moment of birth is clearly marked by the act of departing the womb. In the case of the in vitro fetus, should the equivalent to "birth" be the moment of complete departure from the artificial womb? If so, there is the potential for an anomalous situation in which a prematurely born neonate maintained on a life support system is considered born, whereas an in vitro fetus at the same stage of development and sustained in the same manner is not "born" yet.

Does this mean that in terms of human subject research regulation the in vitro fetus should receive more protection due to the fact that it exists outside of a physical body, and thus "on its own" as a living human? Moreover, considering that the in vitro fetus is no longer protected by the natural shield of a female womb, it is further exposed to the scientific hunger for research than the in vivo fetus. Does this make the in vitro fetus a distinct member of a much more vulnerable class of beings that require extended protection?

The artificial womb requires consideration of the question of how the in vitro fetus should be considered and treated in the eyes of human subject research. Does its unique independent nature and vulnerability require greater protection? What protection is appropriate and at what stage? Inevitably, these questions cannot be answered unless we clarify the moral status of the in vitro fetus. Important questions include: Is an in vitro fetus less than a human person, like a human person or fully a human person? Should it be distinguished from an in vivo fetus? Is its moral status static during the entire gestation, or does its moral status increase according to developmental stages?

A. Equal Moral Status to Equal Development

We believe that the moral status of the in vitro fetus must be equal to that of the in vivo fetus. The mere fact that a fetus is growing externally should not carry any moral weight that decreases our perception of its status. The in vitro fetus is implanted in the AW and begins the process of development toward eventual birth as a human infant, exactly like its fellow in utero. A fetus is a fetus, regardless of its whereabouts and the method of gestation it experiences.

Equal moral value implies that we classify both fetuses in the same category for the purpose of protection from research. Therefore, the definition of this category should include any unborn entity, which is implanted in a human or an artificial womb. Also, it should cover the entire period of gestation, internal or external, up to the point of birth by either exiting a womb or, in external gestation, reaching a stage of fetal development that will be determined.

B. The Need for a Dynamic Moral Status

What should the shared moral status be? Today, in the context of human subject research guidelines and regulations, the moral status of the in vivo fetus is static. That means that it stays the same during the entire gestation period, regardless of the fetus's developmental stages. A two week old in utero embryo is morally equal to a thirty week old fetus. However, it is hard to imagine a static moral status applied in the context of an in vitro fetus. The ability to observe development will compel us to adopt a dynamic approach, which reflects fetal development, in determining the moral status of the in vitro fetus. And it must be dynamic. In other words, the moral status of a fetus must gradually increase as the fetus's development progresses.

There are two main reasons why a dynamic approach is required. The first is the ability to observe fetal development, and the second is the need to balance legal rights in relation to fetuses, such as in the case of abortion.

C. The Ability to Externally Observe Development

The ability to externally observe development inevitably has a tremendous impact on the issue of moral status. The IVF is illustrative of this point. Before IVF it was practically impossible to observe the development of a human embryo. In the traditional, or natural, course of events the initial stages of human embryo development occurred in utero during a period in which a woman was not generally aware that fertilization had actually taken place. The creation of an embryo in a petri dish, external to the body, provided the opportunity to continuously observe human embryonic development. It was, for the first time, accessible and seeable. Observing, externally, the dynamic cell division coupled with the ability to interfere with the process directed focus on a dynamic moral evaluation rather than establishing a static moral definition of an embryo. Moral-biological segmentation into pre-embryo, embryo, primitive streak stage, and establishment of genetic identity, are examples of this dynamic approach.

Similarly, the ability to observe and access a fetus outside the womb will lend a dynamic moral quality to our perception of its developmental stages. Although much research has been done on fetal gestation, we have not yet been able to directly and continuously observe development of the fetus from implantation to birth. Even using the variety of new observation technologies, such as fiber optic photography, thermocameras, ultrasound, and computer generated imaging, the womb is still a fundamental barrier to the accessibility to, and observability of, the fetus.

It is today virtually impossible to have constant accessibility to a pregnant woman's body to observe what is happening within it. Perhaps the biggest challenge the artificial womb presents in this context is that it will cause us to rethink the abstract and arbitrary points that were chosen for the purposes of determining the moral status of an unborn entity. We think there will be a dramatic change in the way scientists, and society in general, will pinpoint the crucial stages of early development. As the medical horizons expand so will the moral debate regarding what we observe. Scientific, moral and legal attention may very well shift to the new visible gestational stages (such as development of organs, organ interconnectivity, brain and nerve activity, and even fetal behavior). This new understanding of fetal development will require a flexible approach to establish moral status.

The ability to externally observe fetal development will have an important psychological effect on the meaning we apply to the developmental stages. It is inescapable that when we evaluate the moral status of an unborn entity, we pay a lot of attention to the extent a developing unborn entity is recognizably human. We naturally attribute moral weight to those beings that physically and behaviorally resemble us. We will become more sympathetic and attribute greater moral value to a fetus, growing in a glass tank, as it gains the shape of a human being. The following is an example of how a fetal body gains a higher moral status once it achieves a recognizably human character: A North Carolina statute providing for the manner of disposition of "remains of pregnancies" requires that the remains of *a recognizable fetus* must be disposed of only by burial or cremation. If not recognizable the remains may be disposed of by generally approved hospital type of incineration.[13]

D. The Need to Balance Conflicting Legal Rights

In addition to the external access and visibility factors, we think that a developmental attitude regarding the moral status of the in vitro fetus will become necessary in order to balance conflicting legal interests in relation to the fetus. Two important legal situations will force us to segment the moral status of the in vitro fetus according to development. One is abortion, and the other is medical malpractice.

As stated earlier, the moral status and standard for human subject research involving in utero fetuses is static throughout the gestation. However, in the context of abortion, the gestation period is distinctly divided into gradual moral standards based upon fetal development or, at least from the legal perspective, the scale of viability. The need to establish a legal decision about abortion rights brought about the need to segment the moral status of the fetus.

The artificial womb will reopen the dilemma of abortion as soon as some one decides to end the life of the fetus by shutting off the gestation machine. The question then will be whether current abortion laws govern in vitro abortion. If not, we will have to consider at what point of development we should allow abortion, which of course includes reestablishing moral status.

With respect to medical malpractice, wrongful or negligent acts by medical teams in relation to the in vitro fetus may result in various malpractice and negligence lawsuits. Today standing to sue is generally granted only to a live born child. However, this may change as the in vitro fetus could be considered "born" earlier and therefore acquire standing to sue while still in the AW, similar to an infant in an incubator. In these cases, and in order to establish the standard of care afforded to the in vitro fetus, the central judicial inquiry would be the stage of development, and the corresponding relevant moral status, in which the wrongful act occurred.

In summary, we think that equal moral status should be applied to both kinds of fetuses. In addition, we believe that the moral status attributed to both should be dynamic and gradual in order to reflect fetal development. New segmentation points will have to be spotted as the ability to externally observe the development increases.

Despite our belief that both in vitro and in vivo fetuses share the same moral status and are to be equally valued, we recognize that additional ethical considerations will be necessary regarding research with an in vivo fetus due to the fact that such research might impact a pregnant woman's health. This means that in some instances research will be allowed with in vitro fetuses that may not be allowed with in vivo fetuses. This does not mean that the moral status of the in vivo fetus is inherently higher. An in vivo fetus should not enjoy more moral weight merely because of its physical connection to a pregnant woman. Thus, whenever research on an in vivo fetus will not affect the pregnant woman, or when the effect is minimal, the same standard must be applied to both kinds of fetuses.

3. Is the AW an Acceptable Medical Procedure?

The moral status of the in vitro fetus is one element in the ethical decision of whether to allow research on fetuses in conjunction with the artificial womb. The other element in that decision is the nature of the research itself. This element includes consideration of the purpose for which this technology would be used, the circumstances in which it would be used, and the scientific manner in which it would be used.

In this section, we will focus on use of the artificial womb for reproductive purposes, and discuss its ethical acceptability solely on that basis. As a framework for this discussion we will review two basic distinctions which have been established in the field so far: the first is the distinction between practice and research and the second is the distinction between therapeutic and non-therapeutic research.

A. The Distinction between Medical Practice and Medical Research

The distinction between medical practice and medical research is one of purpose. The term practice generally refers to intervention designed solely to provide diagnosis, treatment or therapy to an individual patient. Research, on the other hand, designates an activity designed to test a hypothesis and thereby develop or contribute to generalizable knowledge[14] and involves a formal protocol that sets forth an objective and a set of procedures designed to reach that objective.[15] Federal regulations require that any federally funded research, as opposed to medical practice, with human subjects must be examined and approved by an institutional review board (IRB), whose determination should include inquiry into the ethical acceptability of the research.[16]

While research usually exercises new methods and treatments, medical practice usually involves the use of existing knowledge and a routine process with a reasonable expectation of success. The distinction between practice and research is important because the requirements relating to informed consent by the subject of research are generally more stringent than those for practice treatment, and a higher standard of care applies in research to ensure that the potential risk to the subject does not outweigh the potential benefit of the research. However, as the drafters of the Belmont Report noted, the distinction between practice and research is sometimes blurred because both often occur together in a case where treatment becomes experimental. Nonetheless, the fact that a procedure or treatment is experimental in the sense of new, untested, or different, does not automatically place it in the category of research.

B. The Distinction between Therapeutic and Non-therapeutic Research

In the field of research a significant distinction is often made as to whether the research is therapeutic or non-therapeutic. Therapeutic research is for the immediate benefit of the subject whereas non-therapeutic research does not benefit the particular subject but rather benefits other sufferers of the same condition, improves society's medical knowledge, or even benefits the subject at a later date.

This distinction is not one of purpose but of result. It is important to note that the benefit to the subject, in the case of therapeutic research, is not the goal but is a "side effect." Non-therapeutic research usually requires a higher level of ethical justification than therapeutic research, especially when it involves a high risk to the subject's health. However, many researches include both elements and in some cases the distinction is practically imperceptible.

C. Application of the Distinctions to the Artificial Womb

In the case where an artificial womb is used for reproductive purposes to gestate a fetus to birth, is the use of the technology considered practice or research? On one hand, AW falls within the scope of infertility treatment. Because the purpose is to assist individuals who are either unable to conceive or to carry to term, the technology could be categorized as a medical practice. On the other hand, since the technology involves such a drastic departure from the current routine procedures of infertility treatments it would be hard to consider it as an accepted medical practice. This is exactly the type of situation anticipated by the drafters of the Belmont report who recommended that when radically new procedures are used they should be made the object of formal research in the early stages in order to determine whether they are safe and effective.

The acceptability of research with the AW will depend on the progress in the development of the technology over time. Naturally, as the technology is tested and used more frequently, the confusion as to whether it is practice or research will diminish. In this regard, there will be three distinct phases to the technological development that we should consider: the non-therapeutic research phase, the hybrid phase between therapeutic research and practice, and the final phase of pure practice.

D. The Non-therapeutic Research Phase

Today, the AW is a developing technology not yet available as a medical treatment. At present, two scientific teams are conducting research on the development of a reproductive AW. At Cornell University in the United States, a group of scientists are working on prototype wombs created by using cells taken from the endometrial tissue lining the uterus.[17] To date, using hormones and nutrients the tissue has been grown around a dissolvable framework shaped like a uterus. In this research leftover IVF embryos were put into the womb structures and they attached to the walls of the created womb and began to develop. The ultimate goal is to help women who have difficulty conceiving because they have damaged wombs. It is anticipated that the artificial womb, made of a woman's own cells, could be transplanted into her body with little risk of rejection. Another team of scientists at Juntendo University in Japan is approaching the artificial womb from a different perspective. They have taken fetuses from goats and moved them to a rectangular clear plastic box filled with amniotic fluid at body temperature and connected the umbilical cords of the goats to machines which replace oxygen, provide nutrients and eliminate waste. They have been able to sustain fetal goats in this environment for three weeks. The purpose of this research is to help women who have recurrent miscarriages or very premature births.[18] Unlike the Cornell model, which is designed to provide temporary external gestation until re-implantation in the body (partial ectogenesis), the Japanese model of AW is intended to provide full and complete external gestation until birth (complete ectogenesis).

Both scientific teams have shared their projection that the application of AW technology as a practical medical treatment for humans will require much further research, however will be available within this decade. As a practical matter, in this period of technological development, AW is totally experimental. In this phase, scientists will focus on achieving as much medical knowledge as possible about external pregnancy, and therefore that activity should be considered pure research. It is also categorized as non-therapeutic research because this experimental activity will not benefit any particular subject. From the perspective of human subject research guidelines, the utilization of a human fetus for non-therapeutic research should not be allowed if the risk to the fetus is more than minimal, even if the knowledge to be gained is important and cannot be obtained by other means. In this phase, since the risk that the fetus may not survive is great, it would seem that use of human fetuses will not be allowed. Research in this stage must be limited to experiments with animals.

This presents a catch-22 situation. Inevitably, it is the research with humans that is necessary to make AW practicable for humans. It is hard to imagine that the technology can be improved and become safe enough to be used for human fetuses without using human fetuses for that research.

There are at least three situations which we believe would justify the use of AW even at this early stage of technological development. One is when a woman is dying, for example as the result of an accident, and an early development stage fetus would necessarily die if not transferred to an AW. Another is when the mother will die if the pregnancy continues and the fetus is not sufficiently developed to benefit from the use of current neonatal life sustaining equipment. A third situation is when there is a severe medical problem with the fetus itself and in vivo treatment is not possible.

In all the above situations the ethical justification to transfer a human fetus to an experimental artificial womb, despite the high risk, is that using the technology is the only chance to save the fetus's life. In these cases, the use of artificial womb would be considered therapeutic and life saving, even though highly risky. We believe that these extreme circumstances will pave the way for use of human fetuses for the development of the AW at this stage.

E. The Hybrid Phase of Therapeutic Research

Suppose enough knowledge and experience is gained to allow the use of the technology as an established medical treatment for infertility. How would the guidelines apply to such use? Certainly, in the beginning, such a use would still be so innovative that the line between practice and therapeutic research would not be clear. One assumes that in each case where AW is used there will always be research elements aiming to improve the technology and go beyond the limited scope of treatment for the specific patient. In this phase we recommend that, because of the immediacy of the circumstances in any case where an AW might be employed should be examined and reviewed on a case-by-case basis by a hospital's internal ethics committee. For example, the committee should determine in each case what clinical applications of the technology are considered medical practice, and what new experimental elements for research are introduced. Additionally, it is important to consider how beneficial and therapeutic the new experimental elements are, and to whom.

F. Practice

It is easily foreseeable that ten years from now the AW will be a conventional clinical practice offering minimal risks. AW treatment would be as popular as IVF infertility treatment or today's use of neonatal life supporting machines. At this phase, use of the technology would not be a relevant issue for guidelines governing human subject research. However, we do believe that AW technology will remain an infrastructure, and a key method, for various kinds of future fetal research, including gaining general knowledge about fetal development, the etiology and treatment of conditions and diseases, genetic engineering and a variety of medical and scientific inquiries, some of which researchers have yet to imagine. In all those scientific explorations, the usual guidelines must apply as they do today.

The inevitable and undeniable scientific interest in the AW technology, even today, raises another important issue of concern: Will we allow the use of AW for the purpose of research per se?

4. Is the Use of the Artificial Womb for Research Ethically Permissible?

Increasingly, the developments in reproductive technologies open up not only the prospect of improved treatment for infertility, but also a great interest in other medical fields. Embryonic research, which resulted from the IVF technology, is one of the most promising areas of medical research today and brings the potential for identifying and treating many incurable, debilitating and life-threatening illnesses. However, the research on IVF embryos is currently limited to the natural life span of a non implanted embryo. In a lab, after reaching the blastocyst stage of development (maximum 14 days of development), the embryo will expire. Scientists predict that research on more mature embryos, beyond that stage, will provide a tremendous opportunity to learn much more about fetal development, both normal and abnormal. Particular areas of research which interest scientists include mature tissue differentiation, construction of organs and the promise of useful regenerative medicine such as tissue transplantation and gene therapy. Researchers have found that fetal cells divide much faster than adult cells commonly used to engineer tissues.

With such medical promise, it is inevitable that scientists will attempt to culture embryos beyond the blastocyst stage of development, by implantation in animals, by advances in sustaining nascent human life in vitro, or in any form of AW. In this sense, a womb-like apparatus that will keep a fetus externally alive at any stage of development and for any period of time would be considered a form of artificial womb. Due to this strong non-reproductive interest in research we expect these scientific attempts to arise at the very beginning of the technology, even before reproductive application.

The use of AW technology for research per se means that scientists will implant IVF embryos or living aborted fetuses in AW for the sole purpose of research with no intention to bring the fetus to term. Therefore, at some point of the research, the researchers will destroy the in vitro fetus, if it has not expired already as a consequence of the research. When research per se necessarily results in the destruction of the unborn entity, we also refer to it as "destructive research."

How would the ethical regulations and guidelines regarding human subject research impact on this kind of research activity conducted with in vitro fetuses? Is this type of research acceptable? We may learn more about this question from the current approach to research with IVF embryos and living aborted fetuses.

A. Research per se with IVF Embryos

As mentioned before, it is the invention of the IVF treatment in late 1970s that allowed creation of human embryos externally. During the past three decades couples undergoing IVF treatment have consented to donate unused frozen embryos for research, thereby creating the main source for embryos to be used for research per se. Originally only minor restrictions were placed on research involving these donated frozen embryos, and scientists were relatively free to study the embryos. Perhaps the only significant guideline that governed that research was the 14 day rule. As noted previously, many commissions in various countries considered the ethical implications of using such embryos for research and concluded that research should be limited to approximately fourteen days of development. In the United States, this limit was adopted by the National Institute of Health in connection with the most celebrated research using frozen embryos, stem cell research.[18] For although research on embryos is not limited to this application, stem cell research has received attention sufficient to engage the interest of the public and to eclipse discussion of other research using frozen embryos.

Research with human embryos gained enormous public attention after the success of isolating embryonic stem cells in the late 1990s. The acclaimed medical potential of these master cells, derived from the embryo, suddenly put those embryos in the spotlight stirring continuous public debate as to the moral and legal implications of embryonic research.

Stem cell research is a pure form of research per se because it is considered to destroy the embryo. It is a classic case of research per se. Although stem cell research is only one form of research involving embryos, the debate has grown to such proportions that it seems the resolution of this particular issue will determine the whole picture of research with embryos in general.

It is this single consideration—the destruction of the embryo—that drives the debate; and the state of stem cell research, involving the use of frozen embryos, is uncertain. In addition to the 14 day rule, the President of the U.S. by executive order on 9 August 2001 declared federal funding for stem cell research would be limited to then-existing lines of stem cells, and no funding would be provided for research involving use of embryos after that date. However, private funding of such research continues to be possible and California, New Jersey and Massachusetts have all passed state laws encouraging and permitting stem cell research outside the parameters defined by the executive order. Clearly the competing values fueling the public debate have not reached an ultimate resolution. But, the determination of what research is permissible with embryos in stem cell research field will have a significant impact on what research will be permissible regarding development of an artificial womb, specifically implantation of human embryos in AW for the purpose of research.

B. Research per se with Living Aborted Fetuses

Before IVF, the only source of "subjects" available for research on externally living unborn beings was living aborted fetuses. The fact that living aborted fetuses could not exist outside the womb and died very soon, limited that research. Therefore, much scientific effort was directed to maintain them for a longer period in order to allow further research on real-time fetal development.

In the late 1960s, the scientist Dr. Geoffrey Chamberlain worked with living aborted fetuses to conduct his placental research. In his initial experiments he managed to deliver alive a six-month gestational fetus, which was obtained by hysterotomy for therapeutic abortion. Chamberlain placed the aborted fetus in a tank filled with artificial amniotic fluid and connected it to an artificial placenta. The fetus was kept alive for 5 hours and 8 minutes before Chamberlain cut the circuit sustaining the "artificial womb," after which it took 21 minutes for the fetus to expire.[19] Chamberlain's pioneer experiment with living aborted fetus is a precursor of research per se conducted on in vitro fetuses. Would we allow that today?

Currently, statutes in several states prohibit research on living aborted fetuses.[20] These statutes variously define a living fetus as one which displays evidence of a heartbeat, or other obvious signs of life. In such instances no research is permitted until it ceases to show any signs of life. Other states allow research only if "the research is necessary to preserve the life and health of the fetus or child aborted alive."[21] We find the latter legal approach highly interesting because it allows therapeutic research with externally living fetuses that will not survive anyway if no AW is used. Does it imply that any research that extends external fetal life, even for the shortest period, is considered therapeutic and therefore acceptable?

C. Research per se with In Vitro Fetuses

Is research per se with the in vitro fetus acceptable? Compared to research with IVF embryos that are not implanted and would in any case expire naturally after a limited period of time, or research with aborted fetuses, the in vitro fetus can be looked at as a different type of "subject." Growing in an artificial womb, it has the actual potential, rather than philosophic potential, of full development. This alone creates a far more complex ethical situation.

One approach to the question of whether or not we should use in vitro fetuses for research per se is based on the following argument: the artificial womb only creates a potential for growth of those frozen embryos that would otherwise remain in a suspended state indefinitely or be destroyed. In many ways this could be considered like post-mortem organ donation. Similarly, transferring an aborted fetus into an artificial womb for research can be based on the same reasoning. In either instance there is no perceivable loss of life.

A slightly different argument is that to allow what was previously impossible to do for the embryo, to extend life, even for a short period, should be considered therapeutic in the sense that otherwise the embryo would expire earlier. The fact that we terminate the development at a later date is secondary. This argument is supported by the assumption that from the point view of the embryo, it is in "no worse position," and would have chosen to undergo research even if the only benefit is a short period of life. However, the discussion on the dilemma underlying "extend to destroy" situations is beyond the scope of this paper.

One other possible response to this question is to say that the moral status of the in vitro fetuses which are used for research per se is lower than fetuses intended for reproduction. In other words, since these fetuses are not implanted in AW with the intention to bring them to term, they will never become living humans and thus their moral status is lower and the restrictions on using them for research should be minimal. This approach raises the question of how much weight, if any at all, we should give to the intentions of those who implant the in vitro fetus; that is whether the implantation is for therapeutic purposes or not. Should the moral status of an in vitro fetus, implanted purely for research be different from one implanted for reproduction?

We strongly believe that the answer to these questions should be absolutely not. The moral status of an embryo implanted in an AW must not depend on the purpose of the implanters. We believe that this approach to determine moral status is highly dangerous because it implies that we would actually classify life, not on the basis of development, but on the purpose we assign to the unborn entity.

Many people would say there is a wider moral implication of sacrificing an entity with the potential to become part of the human species. How does this reflect on us as a civilized society? (This is a compelling question but must be taken within the context that we also sacrifice existing human lives in wars for ideals.) Indeed, this is the heart of the problem in terms of all research involving human subjects and embryos (which have been consistently viewed by the courts as not humans yet but worthy of being treated with the dignity accorded to the potential to become human). Conceptually, human embryos are a reflection of our own origination, they are what we used to be and they stand for the continuation of our species. We attribute a fair amount of meaning of human life to embryos and fetuses. There is an unconscious survival instinct in us that objects to diminishing the meaning that these entities represent. Thus the concern is always that the value of what a human is will be compromised. To what extent do we allow use of our own kind for the benefit of the larger group?

This brings into play a utilitarian perspective which relies on the benefits gained from the research to outweigh the "cost" of implanting embryos or transferring fetuses into the AW to do research. We do choose, as a society, to make sacrifices if the benefit is agreed to be large enough. Research with in vitro fetuses carries its own benefits to our society. A major benefit of such research would be to increase knowledge of fetal development, understanding genetic deformities, and treating horrible diseases. Other significant benefits would be to allow women who cannot gestate the opportunity to do so without using a surrogate, to protect a developing embryo/fetus from conditions in the womb that may be harmful, and to permit accessibility for corrective surgery to a fetus.

There is no single magic solution applicable to all situations of research per se. AW and the existence of in vitro fetuses will only increase the complexities and expand the dimensions of the dilemma. Nonetheless, we believe that in order to better engage in a meaningful discussion of this dilemma we must first know more about fetal development. Further knowledge will allow us two things: one is to provide a basis to establish a realistic perspective about the moral status of the in vitro fetus; the other is to understand what the gamut of medical opportunities in research with in vitro fetuses is. Based on this knowledge it will make more sense to attempt to establish moral parameters for research.

Our approach to the question of whether or not to use artificial womb as a means of research and using in vitro fetuses for that purpose, is multi-disciplinary. It is rooted in the attempt to establish consistency, to the greatest extent possible, in the moral status valuation of an entity that developmentally is somewhere between a mass of ordinary human cells and a living person. Our approach is to try to reach a unified and coherent ethical landscape that will make sense in conjunction with other aspects of the question. In the case of the AW, we cannot determine the moral status of the in vitro fetus with out keeping in mind the important fact that as a society we already allow abortion.

D. Research per se in relation to abortion

The question whether we should allow research per se with in vitro fetuses and up to what stage of development, if at all, is strongly related to the prospect of terminating the development of an in vitro fetus under the right of abortion. Holding the unified meta-perspective approach we recommend establishing a coordinated protection to the in vitro fetus in both contexts.

The ruling of *Roe v. Wade*[22] established a woman's right to terminate a pregnancy. In this case, the United States Supreme Court also introduced the idea of viability as a tool to measure the moral status of the fetus and thereby the protection it should receive. Viability was there described as the stage of development where the fetus can maintain a "meaningful life out side the mother's womb."[23] The Court developed a trimester framework regarding permissible state regulation of abortion based on its premise that the more developed the fetus is, the greater is the state interest to interfere. Up to the end of the first trimester the right to abort was exclusive, during the second trimester the state's interest increased and at the third trimester, associated with viability, the state's interest was sufficient to prohibit abortion unless continued pregnancy endangered the health of the mother.

Nineteen years after *Roe v. Wade* was decided, the United States Supreme Court in *Planned Parenthood v. Casey*[24] reaffirmed what it held to be *Roe's* central holding that viability marks the earliest point at which the State's interest in fetal life is constitutionally adequate to justify a legislative ban on non-therapeutic abortions. The Court adopted the approach that fetal protection grows according to development towards viability. Moreover, recognizing that with medical advances viability may occur sooner, the Court held the State had an interest in the development of the fetus even before viability.

The above abortion rulings indicate a consistent approach to the question of terminating fetal development, which must be addressed, compared and perhaps adopted by the field of research. How would the idea of fetal viability apply to research with in vitro fetuses?

The development and use of the AW has a profound impact on the concept of viability. On one hand, the ability to externally gestate might serve to establish viability, technically, at implantation from day one. On the other hand, one may argue that true viability requires a substantial chance that the fetus can maintain an independent life outside the womb. Certainly, from this perspective mere implantation in an AW is not sufficient to establish viability. It would be necessary that scientific and medical evidence tend to prove that at a particular point after implantation the chances of the fetus to complete gestation in the artificial womb are highly probable.

We support the latter approach. Knowledge gained from research required to develop the artificial womb has the potential to create a more refined standard for ascertaining viability. It is important to leave the discussion open regarding when it is medically acceptable to say that the option of the AW will lead to birth. From what stage of external development is that probability substantial? In our opinion, that stage, dynamic by definition, should apply both to abortion and to terminating external fetal development for research per se. Once viability is proven, the federal regulations regarding research with fetuses should apply equally to both in vitro and in uterus fetuses. Today the regulations protect the fetus from the moment of implantation. This should be accordingly changed to afford protection from the moment of viability.

To summarize, we think that society's interest in life-saving research, involving use of in vitro fetuses, should not be valued less than the right of a woman to terminate pregnancy. Both purposes are highly important. We may reach the point that AW research conducted before substantial viability occurs, could provide extraordinary benefit to society, would it not be consistent to allow research up to that point?

5. Conclusions

The core dilemma in the field of human subject research is the conflict between the risk to the human subject on the one hand, and the benefit to society from the research on the other. Assisted reproductive technologies have presented a new medium, a new dimension, to this traditional dilemma. They shift the focus from the question of what protection should we afford to a human subject to the new question of what a human subject is.

The prospect of the AW and the possibility of in vitro fetuses will also challenge the question of what a human subject is, but this time to a much greater extent. The AW will bring into the discussion three totally new elements that will change immediately our perception of the development of an unborn human entity. The first element is that the in vitro fetus is separate and independent from a living human body. The second element is that we can observe it becoming physically more recognizably human. The third element is that the in vitro fetus is completely accessible for research.

These three new elements involved in AW technologies will force us not just to decide the moral value of the "new kind" of fetuses, but also we will have to reassess the way we currently value the moral status of in vivo fetuses. If existence within a womb is the only difference between the two fetuses, then that difference cannot justify ethical discrimination. We strongly believe that one clear moral value should apply to both kinds of fetuses. Otherwise, we will open the door to undesirable inconsistency and illogical contradiction.

Moreover, our conclusion is that the moral status of both fetuses must be dynamic in the sense that the moral status increases according to the development of the fetus. But also, in determining this moral value we must make a choice that fits a variety of contexts in which we encounter this entity, such as in the matter of abortion. The determination of a fetus's moral status must make sense in each context individually and in all of them together.

We suggest importing the concept of viability, initially related to abortion, as a key element in determining the moral status of a fetus in general and in the context of human subject research in particular. We also recommend giving the concept of viability more adequate and relevant factors. "Viability" in the context of court decisions is a legal fiction created by the courts to resolve the issue of the legal status of a developing fetus. The definition used, the ability to exist outside the womb albeit with artificial means, becomes practically meaningless with the AW for one main reason: the in vitro fetus already exists outside the womb with artificial means. As soon as an embryo is transferred, implanted, in an AW—an artificial means—it becomes viable under the legal fiction definition. But no one would truly consider this state reflective of the common understanding of viability.

A better definition of viability should be more substantial and include new factors of development that will be studied and become measurable with AW. The level of development of the organs as well as the interconnectivity and function of the system should be assessed to a greater depth of understanding. Also, a level of cognition and observable behavior that evidences such fetal cognition would add dimension to the concept of substantial viability. The question would not be in a womb or not; the main focus of the question would be how recognizably "human" the fetus is. It is probable that with the AW more factors to include in this determination would arise. Research with fetuses growing in AW could be allowed up to the point of substantial viability. Up to this point of development the moral status of a fetus, in vitro or in vivo, deserves respect but only at a minimal level. After substantial viability, which will likely occur sooner and sooner as assisted reproductive technologies develop, the current federal regulations regarding fetal research should apply.

NOTES

1. Nuremberg Code, Directives for Human Experimentation, Reprinted from *Trials of War Criminals before the Nuremberg Military Tribunals under Control Council Law no.* 10, vol. 2 (Washington, D.C.: U.S. Government Printing Office, 1949), pp. 181–182.

2. 18th WMA General Assembly, Helsinki, Finland, June, 1964.

3. Point 6, revised declaration of the 52nd General Assembly, Edinburgh, Scotland, October 2000.

4. Mary Warnock, *A Question of Life: The Warnock Report on Human Fertilisation and Embryology* (Oxford: Blackwell, 1985).

5. *Ibid.*, pp. 58–69.

6. *Ibid.*, p. 66.

7. Karen Dawson, "Segmentation and Moral Status: A Scientific Perspective," in *Embryo Experimentation*, ed. Peter Singer et al. (Cambridge, UK: Cambridge University Press, 1990), pp. 53–64.

8. 93 S.Ct. 705, 35 L.Ed.2d 147, (SC 1973).

9. 45 CFR Part 46.

10. 45 CFR Section 46.204(b).

11. 45 CFR Section 46.202(c).

12. *Roe v. Wade*, 93 S.Ct. 705, 732, 35 L.Ed.2d 147, 163 (SC 1973), New Mexico Statutes, 24-9A-1A: Florida Statutes, 390.0111(4): Wyoming Statutes, 35-6-101(vii).

13. North Carolina Statutes, Section 130A-131.10, "Manner of dispositions of remains in pregnancies."

14. 45 CFR Section 46.102(d).

15. *The Belmont Report: Ethical Principles and Guidelines for the Protection of Human Subjects Research*, The National Commission for the Protection of Human Subjects of Biomedical and Behavioral Research, April 18, 1979 (Washington, D.C.: Government Printing Office, 1979), Part A: Boundaries Between Practice and Research.

16. *NIH Guidelines for the Conduct of Research Involving Human Subjects*, ohsr.od.nih.gov/guidelines/GrayBooklet82404.pdf, sect. 5, p. 10.

16. *Ibid.*

17. Jeremy Rifkin, "The End of Pregnancy," 17 January 2002, *Guardian Unlimited*, http://www.guardian.co.uk/Archive/Article/0,4273,4337092,00.htm; Robin McKie, "Men Redundant? Now We Don't Need Women Either," 10 February 2002, *Guardian Unlimited Observer*, http://observer.guardian.co.uk/international/story/0%2C6903%2C648024%2C00.html.

18. 65 FR 69951, 21 November 2000, updated 11 December 2001, National Institutes of Health Guidelines for Research Using Human Pluripotent Stem Cells, I. Scope of Guidelines.

19. Robert Francoeur, *Utopian Motherhood*, 3rd ed. (New York: Perpetua Books, 1977), pp. 53–55.

20. Massachusetts, MA ST 112 Sec. 12J(a), North Dakota, ND ST Sec. 14-02.2-01, and Rhode Island, RI ST Sec. 11-54-1; California statute, Health and Safety Code, Sec. 123440.

21. Arkansas, AR ST Sec. 20-17-802(b), California, CA HLTH & S, Sec. 123440(a), Missouri, MO ST 188.037.

22. 93 S.Ct. 705, 732, 35 L.Ed.2d 147 (SC 1973).

23. 93 S.Ct. 705, 732, 35 L.Ed.2d 147, 163 (SC 1973).

24. 505 U.S. 833, 112 S.Ct. 2791, 120 L.Ed. 2d 674 (SC 1992).

Thirteen

BIBLIOGRAPHY ON ECTOGENESIS

John R. Shook

Adams, Alice. "Out of the Womb: The Future of the Uterine Metaphor." *Feminist Studies* 19 (1993), pp. 269–289.

Alexander, D. P., et al. "Maintenance of Sheep Fetuses by an Extracorporeal Circuit for Periods up to 24 Hours," *American Journal of Obstetrics and Gynecology* 102 (1968), pp. 969–975.

————. "Maintenance of the Isolated Foetus," *British Medical Bulletin* 22 (1966), pp. 9–12.

————. "Survival of the Foetal Sheep at Term Following Short Periods of Perfusion Through the Umbilical Vessels," *Journal of Physiology* 175 (1964), pp. 113–124.

Angier, Natalie. "Baby in a Box," *New York Times Magazine* (16 May 1999), pp. 86, 88, 90, 154.

Arditti, Rita, Renate Duelli Klein, and Shelley Minden, eds. *Test-Tube Women*. London: Pandora Press, 1984.

Begley, Sharon. "Shaped by Life in the Womb," *Newsweek* 134 (9 September 1999), p. 51.

Bernal, J. D. *The World, the Flesh, and the Devil: An Enquiry into the Future of the Three Enemies of the Rational Soul*. London: Kegan Paul, Trench, and Trubner, 1930.

Brittain, Vera. *Halycyon, or the Future of Monogamy*. London: Kegan Paul, Trench, and Trubner, 1929.

Bulletti, C., et al. "Early Human Pregnancy In Vitro Utilizing an Artificially Perfused Uterus," *Fertility and Sterility* 49 (June 1988), pp. 991–996.

————. "Extracorporeal Perfusion of the Human Uterus." *American Journal of Obstetrics and Gynecology* 154 (March 1986), pp. 683–688.

Buuck, John. "Ethics of Reproductive Engineering," *Perspectives* 3 (1977), pp. 545–547.

184   *JOHN R. SHOOK*

Callaghan, J. C., et al. "Long Term Extracorporeal Circulation in the Development of an Artificial Placenta for Respiratory Distress of the Newborn," *Surgical Forum* 12 (1961), pp. 215–217.

―――. "Studies in the Development of an Artificial Placenta," *Circulation* 27 (1963), pp. 686–690.

―――. "Studies of the First Successful Delivery of an Unborn Lamb after 40 Minutes in the Artificial Placenta," *Canadian Journal of Surgery* 6 (1963), pp. 199–206.

―――. "Studies on Lambs of the Development of an Artificial Placenta," *Canadian Journal of Surgery* 8 (1965), pp. 208–213.

Cannold, Leslie. *The Abortion Myth: Feminism, Morality, and the Hard Choices Women Make*. St. Leonards, N.S.W., Australia: Allen & Unwin, 1998. Middletown, Conn.: Wesleyan University Press, 2001.

―――. "Women, Ectogenesis, and Ethical Theory." *Journal of Applied Philosophy* 12 (1995), pp. 55–64.

―――. "Women's Response to Ectogenesis, and the Relevance of Severance Abortion Theory." Master of Bioethics thesis, Centre for Human Bioethics, Monash University, 1993, supervisor Peter Singer.

―――. "Women's Response to Ectogenesis, Women's Abortion Framework and the Value of Experience to Ethical Theory," in *Philosophy and Applied Ethics Re-Examined* (Newcastle, Australia: University of Newcastle, 1993), pp. 161–174.

Caplan, Arthur. "The Brave New World of Babymaking." *Life* 16 (December 1993), pp. 88–89.

Chamberlain, Geoffrey. "An Artificial Placenta: The Development of an Extra-corporeal System for Maintenance of Immature Infants with Respiratory Problems," *American Journal of Obstetrics and Gynecology* 100 (1968), pp. 615–626.

Coleman, Stephen. "Abortion and the Artificial Womb," *Australasian Journal of Professional and Applied Ethics* 4 (2002), pp. 9–18.

―――. "A Surrogate for Surgery? The Artificial Uterus," *Australasian Journal of Professional and Applied Ethics* 1 (1999), pp. 49–60.

―――. *The Ethics of Artificial Uteruses: Implications for Reproduction and Abortion*. Aldershot, UK: Ashgate, 2004.

Cooper, William. "Placental Chamber—Artificial Uterus," United States Patent number 5,218,958, filed 21 February 1991, granted 15 June 1993; column 1. Cooper's ectogenesis device is described by Sabra Chartrand, "Patents," *New York Times* (19 July 1993), p. D2.

Corea, Gena. *The Mother Machine: Reproductive Technologies from Artificial Insemination to Artificial Wombs.* New York: Harper and Row, 1985.

Corea, Gena, J. Hammer, B. Hoskins, J. Raymond, et al. *Man-made Women: How New Reproductive Technologies Affect Women.* Bloomington: Indiana University Press, 1987.

Donchin, Anne. "The Growing Feminist Debate Over the New Reproductive Technologies," *Hypatia* 4 (1989), pp. 136–149.

Firestone, Shulamith. *The Dialectic of Sex: The Case for Feminist Revolution.* New York: William Morrow and Co., 1970.

Freitas, Robert A., Jr. "Foetal Adoption: A Technological Solution to the Problem of Abortion Ethics," *The Humanist* (May-June 1980), pp. 22–23.

Goodlin, Robert C. "An Improved Fetal Incubator." *Transactions of the American Society for Artificial Internal Organs* 9 (1963), pp. 348–350.

Gosden, Roger. *Designing Babies: The Brave New World of Reproductive Technology.* New York: W. H. Freeman and Co., 1999.

Groeber, Walter R. "Antiabruption Dynamics of the Intervillous Circulation in an Artificial Uterus," *American Journal of Obstetrics and Gynecology* 95 (1966), pp. 640–647.

Grossman, Edward. "The Obsolescent Mother: A Scenario," *The Atlantic* 227 (1971), pp. 39–50.

Hadfield, Peter. "Japanese Pioneers Raise Kid in Rubber Womb," *The New Scientist* (25 April 1992), p. 5.

Haire, Norman. *Hymen, or the Future of Marriage.* London: Kegan Paul, Trench, and Trubner, 1927.

Haldane, Charlotte Franken. *Man's World.* New York: George H. Doran, 1926.

Haldane, J. B. S. *Daedalus, or Science and the Future.* London: Kegan Paul, Trench, Trubner, 1924. Reprinted in *Haldane's Daedalus Revisited*, ed. Krishna R. Dronamraju (Oxford: Oxford University Press, 1995), pp. 23–50.

Harned, H. S., et al. "The Use of the Pump Oxygenator to Sustain Life during Neonatal Asphyxia of Lambs," *AMA Journal of Diseases of Children Society Transactions* 94 (1957), pp. 530–531.

Herlands, Rosalind. "Biological Manipulations for Producing and Nurturing Mammalian Embryos," in *The Custom-Made Child? Women-Centered Perspectives,* eds. Helen B. Holmes, Betty Hoskins, and Michael Gross (Clifton, N.J.: Humana Press, 1981), pp. 231–240.

Huxley, Aldous. *Brave New World: A Novel.* London: Chatto & Windus, 1932. Garden City, N.Y.: Doubleday, Doran, and Co., 1932.

James, David N. "Ectogenesis." In *Encyclopedia of Reproductive Technologies*, ed. Annette Burfoot (Boulder, Col.: Westview, 1999), pp. 370–372.

————. "Ectogenesis: A Reply to Singer and Wells." *Bioethics* 1 (1987), pp. 80–99.

Kamm, Frances Myrna. *Creation and Abortion: An Essay in Moral and Legal Philosophy.* Oxford: Oxford University Press, 1992.

Karp, L. E. "Novel Mechanisms of Reproduction: Preimplantational Ectogenesis," *Postgraduate Medicine* 64 (October 1978), pp. 77–80.

Klass, Perri. "The Artificial Womb is Born." *New York Times Magazine* (29 September 1996), pp. 6–11.

Krantz, K., T. Panos, and J. Evans. "Physiology of the Maternal-Foetal Relationship through the Extracorporeal Circulation of the Human Placenta," *American Journal of Obstetrics and Gynecology* 83 (1962), pp. 1214–1228.

Krever, Horace. "Some Legal Implications of Advances in Human Genetics," *Canadian Journal of Genetics and Cytology* 17 (September 1975), pp. 283–296.

Kuwabara, Yoshinori, et al. "Arterio-venous Extracorporeal Membrane Oxygenation of Fetal Goat Incubated in Artificial Amniotic Fluid (Artificial Placenta): Influence on Lung Growth and Maturation," *Journal of Pediatric Surgery* 33 (1998), pp. 442–448.

————. "Artificial Placenta: Long-Term Extrauterine Incubation of Isolated Goat Fetuses," *Artificial Organs* 13 (1989), pp. 527–531.

————. "Development of an Artificial Placenta: Endocrine Responses of Goat Fetuses during long-term Extrauterine Incubation with Umbilical Arterio-venous Extracorporeal Membrane Oxygenation," *Endocrine Journal* 41 (1994), pp. S69–S76.

————. "Development of an Artificial Placenta: Optimal Extracorporeal Blood Flow in Goat Fetuses during Extrauterine Incubation with Umbilical Arteriovenous Extracorporeal Membrane Oxygenation," *Artificial Organs Today* 2 (1992), pp. 197–204.

————. "Development of an Artificial Placenta: Survival of Isolated Goat Fetuses for Three Weeks with Umbilical Arteriovenous Extracorporeal Membrane Oxygenation," *Artificial Organs* 17 (1993), pp. 996–1003.

————. "Development of Artificial Placenta: Oxygen Metabolism of Isolated Goat Fetuses with Umbilical Arteriovenous Extracorporeal Membrane Oxygenation," *Fetal Diagnosis and Therapy* 5 (1990), pp. 189–195.

————. "Development of an Extrauterine Fetal Incubation System Using an Extracorporeal Membrane Oxygenator," *Artificial Organs* 11 (1987), pp. 224–227.

————. "Goat Fetuses Disconnected from the Placenta, but Reconnected to an Artificial Placenta, Display Intermittent Breathing Movements," *Biology of the Neonate* 75 (1999), pp. 388–397.

————. "Metabolic and Endocrine Responses to Cold Exposure in Chronically-incubated Extrauterine Goat Fetuses," *Pediatric Research* 43 (1998), pp. 452–460.

Lawn, L., and R. A. McCance. "Artificial Placentae: A Progress Report," *Acta Paediatrica* 53 (1964), pp. 317–325.

Liu, Hung-Ching, et al. "Human Preembryo Development on Autologous Endometrial Coculture versus Conventional Medium," *Fertility and Sterility* 70 (1998), pp. 1109–1113.

Ludovici, Anthony M. *Lysistratra, or Woman's Future and Future Woman*. London: Kegan Paul, Trench, and Trubner, 1927.

Lupton, M. L. "Artificial Wombs: Medical Miracle, Legal Nightmare." *Journal of Medical Law* 16 (1997), pp. 621–633.

————. "The Role of the Artificial Uterus in Embryo Adoption and Neonatal Intensive Care," *Medicine and Law* 18 (1999), pp. 613–629.

McDonough, Paul G. (1988) "Comment." *Fertility and Sterility* 50:6 (June) 1001–1002.

McKie, Robin. "Men Redundant? Now We Don't Need Women Either," *Guardian Unlimited Observer* (10 February 2002), http://observer.guardian. co.uk/international/story/0%2C6903%2C648024%2C00.html

Murphy, Julien S. "Abortion Rights and Fetal Termination." *Journal of Social Philosophy* 15 (1989), pp. 11–16.

————. "Is Pregnancy Necessary: Feminist Concerns About Ectogenesis." *Hypatia* 4 (1989), pp. 66–84.

Nixon, D. A., et al. "Perfusion of the Viable Sheep Foetus," *Nature* 199 (1963), pp. 183–185.

————. "Ventures with an Artificial Placenta I. Principles and Preliminary Results," *Proceedings of the Royal Society B* 155 (1962), pp. 500–509.

————. "Artificial Reproduction and the Family of the Future," *Medicine and Law* 17 (1998), pp. 93–111.

Overall, Christine. *Human Reproduction: Principles, Practices, Policies*. Toronto: Oxford University Press, 1993.

Pak, Sok Cheon, et al. "Extrauterine Incubation of Fetal Goats Applying the Extracorporeal Membrane Oxygenation via Umbilical Artery and Vein," *Journal of Korean Medical Science* 17 (2002), pp. 663–668.

Paul, Eden. *Chronos, or the Future of the Family*. London: Kegan Paul, Trench, and Trubner, 1930.

Piercy, Marge. *Women on the Edge of Time*. New York: Alfred A. Knopf, 1976.

The President's Council on Bioethics. *Human Cloning and Human Dignity: An Ethical Inquiry*. Washington, D.C.: The President's Council on Bioethics, 2002.

Purdy, Laura. "The Morality of New Reproductive Technologies," *Journal of Social Philosophy* 18 (Winter 1987), pp. 38–48.

Reuters News Wire, "Japanese Scientist Develops Artificial Womb," (18 July 1997).

Rich, Adrienne. *Of Woman Born: Motherhood as Experience and Institution*. New York: W. W. Norton, 1979.

Rifkin, Jeremy. "The End of Pregnancy," *Guardian Unlimited* (17 January 2002), http://www.guardian.co.uk/Archive/Article/0,4273,4337092,00.html

Robertson, John A. "Procreative Liberty and the Control of Conception, Pregnancy, and Childbirth," *Virginia Law Review* 69 (1983), pp. 405–464.

Rosen, Christine. "Why Not Artificial Wombs?" *The New Atlantis* 3 (Fall 2003), pp. 67–76.

Rowland, Robyn. "Motherhood, Patriarchal Power, Alienation and the Issue of Choice," in *Man-made Women: How New Reproductive Technologies Affect Women*, eds. Gena Corea et al. (London: Hutchinson, 1985; Bloomington: Indiana University Press, 1987), pp. 74–87.

————. "Of Women Born, But for How Long? The Relationship of Women to the New Reproductive Technologies and the Issue of Choice," in *Made to Order: The Myth of Reproductive and Genetic Progress*, eds. Patricia Spallone and Deborah L. Steinberg (Oxford: Pergamon Press, 1987), pp. 67–83.

————. "Reproductive Technologies: The Final Solution to the Woman Question," in *Test-Tube Women: What Future for Motherhood?*, eds. Ruth Arditti, Rebecca Klein, and Shelley Minden (London: Pandora Press, 1984), pp. 356–369.

Sakata, M., K. Hisano, M. Okada, and M. Yasufuku. "A New Artificial Placenta with a Centrifugal Pump: Long-term Total Extrauterine Support of Goat Fetuses," *Journal of Thoracic and Cardiovascular Surgery* 115 (1998), pp. 1023–1031.

Sarin, C. L., et al. "Further Development of an Artificial Placenta with the use of Membrane Oxygenator and Venovenous Perfusion," *Surgery* 60 (1966), pp. 754–760.

SenGupta, A., et al. "An Artificial Placenta Designed to Maintain Life during Cardiovascular Distress," *Transactions: American Society for Artificial Internal Organs* 10 (1964), pp. 63–65.

Silver, Lee M. *Remaking Eden: Cloning and Beyond in a Brave New World.* New York: Avon Books, 1997.

Singer, Peter, and Deane Wells. "Ectogenesis." In *The Reproductive Revolution: New Ways of Making Babies* (Oxford: Oxford University Press, 1984), pp. 131–149. Revised version in *Making Babies: The New Science and Ethics of Conception* (New York: Charles Scribner's Sons, 1985), pp. 116–134.

Squier, Susan Merrill. *Babies in Bottles: Twentieth-Century Visions of Reproductive Technology.* New Brunswick, N.J.: Rutgers University Press, 1994.

Standaert, T. A., et al. "Extracorporeal Support of the Fetal Lamb Simulating in Utero Gas Exchange," *Gynecological Investigations* 5 (1974), pp. 93–105.

Walters, William A. W. "Cloning, Ectogenesis, and Hybrids: Things to Come?" In *Test-Tube Babies: A Guide to Moral Questions, Present Techniques and Future Possibilities*, eds. William Walters and Peter Singer (Melbourne, Australia: Oxford University Press, 1982), pp. 110–118, 157–158.

Warnock, Mary. *A Question of Life: The Warnock Report on Human Fertilization and Embryology.* Oxford: Basil Blackwell, 1984.

Welin, Stellan. "Reproductive Ectogenesis: The Third Era of Human Reproduction and Some Moral Consequences," *Science and Engineering Ethics* 10 (2004), pp. 615–626.

Wells, Deane. "Ectogenesis, Justice, and Utility: A Reply to James." *Bioethics* 1 (1987), pp. 372–379.

Westin, B., et al. "A Technique for Perfusion of the Previable Human Fetus," *Acta Paediatrica* 47 (1958), pp. 339–349.

Zapol, W. M., et al. "Artificial Placenta: Two Days of Total Extrauterine Support of the Isolated Premature Lamb Fetus," *Science* 166 (1969), pp. 617–618.

Zimmerman, Sacha. "Fetal Position." *The New Republic* 229 (18 August 2003), pp. 14, 16–17.

ABOUT THE EDITORS AND CONTRIBUTORS

Jennifer Bard is Associate Professor of Law at Texas Tech University. She has been an Assistant Attorney General in the Connecticut Attorney General's Office and an Associate Member of the Health Law and Policy Institute at the University of Houston. She has published on legal ethics, medical ethics, and reproductive technologies.

Leslie Cannold is a Research Fellow at the Centre for Applied Philosophy and Public Ethics at the University of Melbourne, Australia. She has authored many book chapters and articles on diverse social and ethical issues. She is the author of *The Abortion Myth: Feminism, Morality and the Hard Choices Women Make,* and *What, No Baby: Why Women are Losing the Freedom to Mother, and How They Can Get It Back.*

Scott Gelfand is Associate Professor of Philosophy and Director of the Ethics Center at Oklahoma State University. His publications are in the areas of ethical theory, applied ethics, and political theory.

Dien Ho is Assistant Professor of Philosophy at the University of Kentucky and serves on the Hospital Ethics Committee of the University of Kentucky Hospital. His research interests include medical ethics, liberal theory, and theoretical reasoning.

Nadav Mazor is a biotechnology attorney and the legal counsel for the Human Cloning Foundation. He is a member of the Committee on Bioethical Issues at the Association of the Bar of the City of New York and a member of the Institutional Review Board at New York University. As a visiting international scholar at the Hastings Center he conducted research on the artificial womb.

Julien S. Murphy is founding Director of the Bioethics Project and Professor of Philosophy at the University of Southern Maine. Her many publications include writings in the areas of feminist theory, medical ethics, and recent continental philosophy. She is the editor of *Feminist Interpretations of Jean-Paul Sartre.*

Gregory Pence is Professor in the Philosophy Department and the School of Medicine at the University of Alabama at Birmingham. He is the author of *Classic Cases in Medical Ethics*; *Designer Food: Mutant Harvest or Breadbasket for the World?* and *Cloning after Dolly: Who's Still Afraid?*

Joyce M. Raskin is Project Director of the Louis Stein Center for Law and Ethics at Fordham University School of Law. She has broad legal experience in the areas of products liability, medical malpractice, and environmental concerns. She is a member of the Bioethical Issues Committee of the Association of the Bar of the City of New York and the American Society for Law Medicine and Ethics. She sits on two Institutional Review Boards dealing with research involving human subjects.

Maureen Sander-Staudt is Assistant Professor of Philosophy at Arizona State University, West Campus. Her publications and research presently center on issues in feminism, care ethics, and applied ethics, particularly bioethics, reproductive technologies, and moral education.

John R. Shook is Provost and Senior Research Fellow at the Center for Inquiry Transnational in Amherst, New York. His interests in applied ethics are inspired by his study of American philosophy and pragmatism, and he has published several books relating to these fields.

Peter Singer is DeCamp Professor of Bioethics in the University Center for Human Values at Princeton University. He is the author of books on many topics in ethics, including *Animal Liberation: A New Ethics of Our Treatment of Animals*; *Practical Ethics*; *The Reproduction Revolution: New Ways of Making Babies* with Deane Wells; and *Rethinking Life and Death*.

Rosemarie Tong is Distinguished Professor of Health Care Ethics and the Director of the Center for Professional and Applied Ethics at the University of North Carolina at Charlotte. Tong is the author of many books including *Feminine and Feminist Ethics*; *Controlling Our Reproductive Destiny* with Lawrence Kaplan; *Feminist Approaches to Bioethics*; and *Linking Visions: Feminist Bioethics, Human Rights, and the Developing World*.

Deane Wells is a former Attorney General of Queensland, and he also was a representative to the Australian Parliament during 1983–1984.

Joan Woolfrey is Associate Professor of Philosophy at West Chester University where she pursues her research in biomedical ethics and feminist thought. She has been the co-director of the Pharmaceutical Product Development program at West Chester University.

INDEX

Steptoe, Patrick Christopher, 20
Sterba, James, 111, 127
Stevenson, Patricia A., 74
Suh, Mary, 43, 46
surrogacy, ix, 11, 17, 33, 35, 59,
    62, 66–70, 79–81, 84–87,
    97, 100, 135, 177

Tabanelli, S., 44
Thomson, Judith Jarvis, 49, 58,
    103–104, 107, 152–153, 157
Tong, Rosemarie, 3, 4, 59
Tyson, J. E., 137

utilitarianism, 89, 98, 107, 152–
    153, 177

Vargyas, Joyce, 20
virtue ethics, 90–107

Wagner, Marsden G., 74
Waldschmidt, Anne, 74
Walters, LeRoy, 74
Walters, William A. W., 74, 189
Warnock, Mary, 46, 162, 181, 189
Warnock Report, The (Warnock),
    28, 29, 46, 161, 162, 181,
    189
Warren, Mary Anne, 58, 104, 107
Welin, Stellan, 189
Wells, Deane, 4, 9, 38, 41, 45, 46,
    67–70, 75–76, 147, 186, 189
Wells, Herbert George, 61
Westin, B., 189
Whitehead, Mary Beth, 68, 84
Wilson, James Q., 147
women,
    elimination of w., 36–37,
        134
    liberation of w., 3, 5, 12–14,
        17–19, 27, 29, 34–38,
        60–64, 83, 111–115,
        126, 129–138

power of w., 17, 65, 68,
    111–117, 121–127, 129,
    136, 153
Woolfrey, Joan, 5, 129

Yasufuku, M., 189

Zapol, W. M., 189
Zimmerman, Sacha, 6, 189

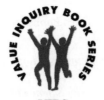

VIBS

The **Value Inquiry Book Series** is co-sponsored by:

Adler School of Professional Psychology
American Indian Philosophy Association
American Maritain Association
American Society for Value Inquiry
Association for Process Philosophy of Education
Canadian Society for Philosophical Practice
Center for Bioethics, University of Turku
Center for Professional and Applied Ethics, University of North Carolina at Charlotte
Central European Pragmatist Forum
Centre for Applied Ethics, Hong Kong Baptist University
Centre for Cultural Research, Aarhus University
Centre for Professional Ethics, University of Central Lancashire
Centre for the Study of Philosophy and Religion, University College of Cape Breton
Centro de Estudos em Filosofia Americana, Brazil
College of Education and Allied Professions, Bowling Green State University
College of Liberal Arts, Rochester Institute of Technology
Concerned Philosophers for Peace
Conference of Philosophical Societies
Department of Moral and Social Philosophy, University of Helsinki
Gannon University
Gilson Society
Haitian Studies Association
Ikeda University
Institute of Philosophy of the High Council of Scientific Research, Spain
International Academy of Philosophy of the Principality of Liechtenstein
International Association of Bioethics
International Center for the Arts, Humanities, and Value Inquiry
International Society for Universal Dialogue
Natural Law Society
Philosophical Society of Finland
Philosophy Born of Struggle Association
Philosophy Seminar, University of Mainz
Pragmatism Archive at The Oklahoma State University
R.S. Hartman Institute for Formal and Applied Axiology
Research Institute, Lakeridge Health Corporation
Russian Philosophical Society
Society for Existential Analysis
Society for Iberian and Latin-American Thought
Society for the Philosophic Study of Genocide and the Holocaust
Unit for Research in Cognitive Neuroscience, Autonomous University of Barcelona
Yves R. Simon Institute

Titles Published

15. Sidney Axinn, *The Logic of Hope: Extensions of Kant's View of Religion*

16. Messay Kebede, *Meaning and Development*

17. Amihud Gilead, *The Platonic Odyssey: A Philosophical-Literary Inquiry into the Phaedo*

18. Necip Fikri Alican, *Mill's Principle of Utility: A Defense of John Stuart Mill's Notorious Proof.* A volume in **Universal Justice**

19. Michael H. Mitias, Editor, *Philosophy and Architecture.*

20. Roger T. Simonds, *Rational Individualism: The Perennial Philosophy of Legal Interpretation.* A volume in **Natural Law Studies**

21. William Pencak, The Conflict of Law and Justice in the Icelandic Sagas

22. Samuel M. Natale and Brian M. Rothschild, Editors, *Values, Work, Education: The Meanings of Work*

23. N. Georgopoulos and Michael Heim, Editors, *Being Human in the Ultimate: Studies in the Thought of John M. Anderson*

24. Robert Wesson and Patricia A. Williams, Editors, *Evolution and Human Values*

25. Wim J. van der Steen, *Facts, Values, and Methodology: A New Approach to Ethics*

26. Avi Sagi and Daniel Statman, *Religion and Morality*

27. Albert William Levi, *The High Road of Humanity: The Seven Ethical Ages of Western Man*, Edited by Donald Phillip Verene and Molly Black Verene

28. Samuel M. Natale and Brian M. Rothschild, Editors, *Work Values: Education, Organization, and Religious Concerns*

29. Laurence F. Bove and Laura Duhan Kaplan, Editors, *From the Eye of the Storm: Regional Conflicts and the Philosophy of Peace.* A volume in **Philosophy of Peace**

30. Robin Attfield, *Value, Obligation, and Meta-Ethics*

46. Peter A. Redpath, *Wisdom's Odyssey: From Philosophy to Transcendental Sophistry.* A volume in **Studies in the History of Western Philosophy**

47. Albert A. Anderson, *Universal Justice: A Dialectical Approach.* A volume in **Universal Justice**

48. Pio Colonnello, *The Philosophy of José Gaos.* Translated from Italian by Peter Cocozzella. Edited by Myra Moss. Introduction by Giovanni Gullace. A volume in **Values in Italian Philosophy**

49. Laura Duhan Kaplan and Laurence F. Bove, Editors, *Philosophical Perspectives on Power and Domination: Theories and Practices.* A volume in **Philosophy of Peace**

50. Gregory F. Mellema, *Collective Responsibility*

51. Josef Seifert, *What Is Life? The Originality, Irreducibility, and Value of Life.* A volume in **Central-European Value Studies**

52. William Gerber, *Anatomy of What We Value Most*

53. Armando Molina, *Our Ways: Values and Character*, Edited by Rem B. Edwards. A volume in **Hartman Institute Axiology Studies**

54. Kathleen J. Wininger, *Nietzsche's Reclamation of Philosophy.* A volume in **Central-European Value Studies**

55. Thomas Magnell, Editor, *Explorations of Value*

56. HPP (Hennie) Lötter, *Injustice, Violence, and Peace: The Case of South Africa.* A volume in **Philosophy of Peace**

57. Lennart Nordenfelt, *Talking About Health: A Philosophical Dialogue.* A volume in **Nordic Value Studies**

58. Jon Mills and Janusz A. Polanowski, *The Ontology of Prejudice.* A volume in **Philosophy and Psychology**

59. Leena Vilkka, *The Intrinsic Value of Nature*

157.   Javier Muguerza, *Ethics and Perplexity: Toward a Critique of Dialogical Reason.* Translated from the Spanish by Jody L. Doran. Edited by John R. Welch. A volume in **Philosophy in Spain**

158.   Gregory F. Mellema, *The Expectations of Morality*

159.   Robert Ginsberg, *The Aesthetics of Ruins*

160.   Stan van Hooft, *Life, Death, and Subjectivity: Moral Sources in Bioethics* A volume in **Values in Bioethics**

161.   André Mineau, *Operation Barbarossa: Ideology and Ethics Against Human Dignity*

162.   Arthur Efron, *Expriencing Tess of the D'Urbervilles: A Deweyan Account.* A volume in **Studies in Pragmatism and Values**

163.   Reyes Mate, *Memory of the West: The Contemporaneity of Forgotten Jewish Thinkers.* Translated from the Spanish by Anne Day Dewey. Edited by John R. Welch. A volume in **Philosophy in Spain**

164.   Nancy Nyquist Potter, Editor, *Putting Peace into Practice: Evaluating Policy on Local and Global Levels.* A volume in **Philosophy of Peace**

165.   Matti Häyry, Tuija Takala, and Peter Herissone-Kelly, Editors, *Bioethics and Social Reality.* A volume in **Values in Bioethics**

166.   Maureen Sie, *Justifying Blame: Why Free Will Matters and Why it Does Not.* A volume in **Studies in Applied Ethics**

167.   Leszek Koczanowicz and Beth J. Singer, Editors, *Democracy and the Post-Totalitarian Experience.* A volume in **Studies in Pragmatism and Values**

168.   Michael W. Riley, *Plato's* Cratylus: *Argument, Form, and Structure.* A volume in **Studies in the History of Western Philosophy**

169.   Leon Pomeroy, *The New Science of Axiological Psychology.* Edited by Rem B. Edwards. A volume in **Hartman Institute Axiology Studies**

170.   Eric Wolf Fried, *Inwardness and Morality*

171.   Sami Pihlstrom, *Pragmatic Moral Realism: A Transcendental Defense.* A volume in Studies in **Pragmatism and Values**

172.   Charles C. Hinkley II, *Moral Conflicts of Organ Retrieval: A Case for Constructive Pluralism*. A volume in **Values in Bioethics**

173.   Gábor Forrai and George Kampis, Editors, *Intentionality: Past and Future*. A volume in **Cognitive Science**

174.   Dixie Lee Harris, *Encounters in My Travels: Thoughts Along the Way*. A volume in **Lived Values:Valued Lives**

175.   Lynda Burns, Editor, *Feminist Alliances*. A volume in **Philosophy and Women**

176.   George Allan and Malcolm D. Evans, *A Different Three Rs for Education*. A volume in **Philosophy of Education**

177.   Robert A. Delfino, Editor, *What are We to Understand Gracia to Mean?*: *Realist Challenges to Metaphysical Neutralism*. A volume in **Gilson Studies**

178.   Constantin V. Ponomareff and Kenneth A. Bryson, *The Curve of the Sacred: An Exploration of Human Spirituality*. A volume in **Philosophy and Religion**

179.   John Ryder, Gert Rüdiger Wegmarshaus, Editors, *Education for a Democratic Society: Central European Pragmatist Forum, Volume Three*. A volume in **Studies in Pragmatism and Values**

180.   Florencia Luna, *Bioethics and Vulnerability: A Latin American View*. A volume in **Values in Bioethics**

181.   John Kultgen and Mary Lenzi, Editors, *Problems for Democracy*. A volume in **Philosophy of Peace**

182.   David Boersema and Katy Gray Brown, Editors, *Spiritual and Political Dimensions of Nonviolence and Peace*. A volume in **Philosophy of Peace**

183.   Daniel P. Thero, *Understanding Moral Weakness*. A volume in **Studies in the History of Western Philosophy**

184.   Scott Gelfand and John R. Shook, Editors, *Ectogenesis: Artificial Womb Technology and the Future of Human Reproduction*. A volume in **Values in Bioethics**